# Variable Resistance Training (VRT): Transforming Strength Training with Resistance Bands

SOUTHERLAND | COPYRIGHT 2023

# Introduction

Welcome to a journey through the innovative world of Variable Resistance Training (VRT), a methodology set to transform the way we approach strength and fitness training. This book is designed to guide you through the nuances of VRT, contrasting it with traditional weight training to unveil a path to enhanced muscle growth, improved flexibility, and reduced risk of injury.

In the realm of fitness and strength training, traditional methods have long dominated the scene, often focusing on fixed resistance through weights. While effective, these methods come with limitations, including the risk of plateaus and a higher likelihood of injury. Variable Resistance Training emerges as a dynamic alternative, introducing an adaptable approach to strength training that aligns with the body's natural strength curves and capabilities.

Throughout this book, we delve into the core principles of VRT, exploring the science behind why and how it works. We examine the limitations of conventional weight training, highlighting how VRT offers a safer and more efficient pathway to achieving your strength and fitness goals. With a detailed look at various types of VRT equipment, from simple resistance bands to sophisticated machines, we open up a world of possibilities for enhancing your workout regimen.

Practical application forms a cornerstone of this book. Detailed chapters provide guidance on creating personalized VRT programs, considering different fitness levels and objectives. We cover a range of exercises, complete with setup and execution instructions, showing you how to incorporate VRT into your routine effectively.

But this book is more than just a guide to exercises. It's a comprehensive approach to training, emphasizing the importance of listening to your body, making necessary adjustments, and understanding the critical role of recovery and maintenance in your fitness journey.

Whether you're a fitness enthusiast looking to elevate your workout, a beginner seeking a safe entry into strength training, or an athlete aiming for peak performance, this book is your companion to a more effective, fulfilling, and injury-free approach to fitness. Let's embark on this journey together, redefining resistance and unlocking the full potential of your strength training endeavors.

## Variable Resistance Training

Variable Resistance Training (VRT) is an innovative approach in strength and fitness training that diverges from traditional weightlifting methods. At its core, VRT involves the use of equipment or techniques that modify the resistance throughout the range of motion in an exercise. Unlike conventional weights that maintain a constant load, variable resistance adapts, typically increasing where the muscles are strongest and decreasing where they are weakest.

The primary mechanism behind VRT is to align the resistance with the natural strength curves of muscles. Muscles have varying degrees of strength at different points in their range of motion. VRT takes advantage of this by altering the resistance to match these fluctuations in strength. This is often achieved through equipment like resistance bands, adjustable resistance machines, or even modified free weights.

Benefits Over Traditional Weight Training

- Enhanced Muscle Activation: By varying resistance, VRT can lead to more comprehensive muscle activation as it challenges muscles at their strongest points.

- Reduced Risk of Injury: Traditional weights can place excessive strain on muscles and joints at their weakest points. VRT minimizes this risk by reducing load where the body is most vulnerable.

- Overcoming Plateaus: Standard weightlifting can lead to performance plateaus. VRT, with its changing resistance, continually challenges the muscles, promoting sustained progress.

VRT in Practice

In practice, VRT is not limited to specialized equipment. It can be as simple as attaching resistance bands to free weights or using machines that automatically adjust resistance. The key is the variation in load throughout an exercise, which can lead to more dynamic and effective workouts.

Variable Resistance Training represents a significant shift in how we approach strength training. It's not just about lifting weights; it's about understanding and working with the body's natural strengths and weaknesses to achieve more efficient and safer workouts. This introduction sets the stage for a deeper exploration of VRT's principles, applications, and benefits in subsequent chapters.

# Brief Contrast with Traditional Weight Training

While Variable Resistance Training (VRT) and traditional weight training are both aimed at improving strength and fitness, they differ fundamentally in their approach and execution. Understanding these differences is key to appreciating the unique advantages of VRT.

Traditional Weight Training

- Constant Resistance: In traditional weight training, the resistance (weight of the dumbbell, barbell, or machine) remains constant throughout the movement. This means that the muscle experiences the same load in both its strongest and weakest points in the range of motion.

- Muscle Activation: Traditional methods often focus on specific muscle groups and may not engage supporting or stabilizing muscles to the same extent as VRT.

- Risk of Injury: Due to constant resistance, there's a potential risk of injury, especially when lifting heavy weights, as the joints and muscles are under consistent strain throughout the movement.

- Plateauing: Users of traditional weight training might experience plateaus in strength and muscle development, as the muscles get accustomed to the consistent load.

Variable Resistance Training

- Dynamic Resistance: VRT changes the resistance at different phases of an exercise. This aligns better with the muscle's natural strength curve, offering less resistance where the muscle is weakest and more where it's strongest.

- Holistic Muscle Engagement: VRT tends to engage more muscle fibers, including stabilizing muscles, due to the varying resistance, leading to more balanced muscle development.

- Reduced Injury Risk: By reducing resistance at weaker points in a movement, VRT minimizes the strain on joints and muscles, potentially lowering the risk of injury.

- Overcoming Plateaus: The varying resistance in VRT can prevent muscle adaptation, continuously challenging muscles and thus helping to avoid performance plateaus.

# Analysis Of The Plateau Effect In Weight Training

The plateau effect in weight training is a common challenge faced by many individuals engaged in regular strength training routines. This phenomenon occurs when a person experiences a noticeable slowdown or complete halt in workout progress, particularly in terms of strength gains, muscle growth, or weight loss. In traditional weight training, where exercises involve lifting a constant weight, the muscles adapt to the specific demands placed on them over time. This adaptation, while initially beneficial, can lead to a point where the muscles no longer find the same level of resistance challenging.

One of the primary reasons for hitting a plateau is the body's remarkable ability to become efficient at performing repeated tasks. When the same exercises with the same weight and repetition scheme are continually performed, the muscles become very efficient at executing these movements, reducing the overall effectiveness of the workout. This efficiency, while a natural and impressive feature of the human body, can hinder progress in strength training.

Another contributing factor is the lack of variation in traditional weight training routines. Without changes in exercise selection, weight, repetitions, and other training variables, the stimulus provided to the muscles remains too consistent, leading to diminished returns over time. In addition to physical factors, plateaus can also be influenced by nutritional and recovery aspects. Adequate nutrition and rest are crucial for muscle growth and strength improvements. Neglecting these can impede progress, contributing to the plateau effect.

To overcome this plateau, trainers often recommend altering workout routines by increasing the weight, changing the number of repetitions, varying the exercises, or incorporating different types of training like high-intensity interval training (HIIT) or plyometrics. These changes can provide new challenges to the muscles, forcing them to adapt and grow. In the context of variable resistance training, the changing resistance throughout an exercise can naturally counteract the plateau effect. By continuously varying the resistance, the muscles are constantly challenged in new ways, making it harder for them to become fully adapted and efficient at any given exercise, thus potentially maintaining progress and growth over a more extended period.

## The Risk Of Injuries Associated With Traditional Weights

The use of traditional weights in strength training, while effective for muscle building and fitness improvement, carries a risk of injuries. These injuries can range from acute trauma, such as strains or sprains, to long-term issues like joint wear and tear or chronic pain. One of the primary reasons for these risks is the nature of the constant load that traditional weights impose on the body. When lifting a fixed weight, especially if it's heavy, the muscles, tendons, and joints consistently bear the same load throughout the exercise movement. This can put undue stress on specific areas, particularly if the lifter's technique is not optimal or if the body is not adequately prepared for the load.

Another injury risk factor is the potential for overuse injuries. These occur when the same movements are repeated frequently over time, leading to strain on specific muscles and joints. Such repetitive stress, without adequate rest and recovery, can lead to conditions like tendonitis or stress fractures. Traditional weight training can also place disproportionate stress on the lower back, shoulders, and knees. These areas are often susceptible to injury due to the high loads they bear in exercises like squats, deadlifts, and bench presses.

Poor form and technique significantly contribute to the risk of injury. Lifting weights that are too heavy or performing exercises with incorrect form can lead to acute injuries like muscle tears or herniated discs. Additionally, the lack of variability in traditional weight training can contribute to muscular imbalances, where certain muscles become stronger while others remain underdeveloped. This imbalance can lead to poor posture and increased susceptibility to injury.

To mitigate these risks, it's essential to focus on proper technique, start with manageable weights, and gradually increase the load. Including a variety of exercises in the training regimen can help in developing balanced muscle strength and reducing the risk of overuse injuries. Rest and recovery, along with proper nutrition, play a crucial role in injury prevention. Moreover, incorporating training methods like variable resistance can offer a safer alternative by aligning the resistance with the body's natural strength curves, reducing the load where the body is weakest and potentially decreasing the risk of injury.

# Scientific Studies Showing Limitations Of Fixed Resistance

Scientific studies in the field of exercise physiology and sports science have explored the limitations of fixed resistance in traditional weight training. These studies have provided valuable insights into how constant loads can sometimes be less effective or potentially riskier compared to variable resistance methods.

One key area of research focuses on muscle activation and growth. Studies have shown that fixed resistance does not always optimally activate muscles throughout the entire range of motion. Since the resistance does not change, it may not effectively target muscle fibers at their strongest points, potentially leading to less efficient muscle growth. This is particularly evident in exercises where the muscle's leverage changes significantly, such as in squats or bench presses. In these movements, certain portions of the exercise can be relatively easy, while others might be extremely challenging, leading to uneven muscle development.

Another significant area of study is the risk of injury associated with fixed resistance training. Research has indicated that the constant load of traditional weights can put undue stress on joints and connective tissues. This is especially true for exercises that place a high load on the body in positions where muscles and joints are at their weakest, increasing the risk of strains, sprains, and chronic joint issues. For example, in exercises like the deadlift or squat, the lower back can be particularly vulnerable if the weight is too heavy or the form is improper.

Furthermore, studies have also highlighted the issue of training plateaus with fixed resistance. Muscle adaptation is a well-documented phenomenon where muscles become more efficient at handling a specific load if it's repeatedly used over time. This efficiency, while beneficial to some degree, can lead to a plateau in muscle growth and strength gains. The muscle no longer finds the resistance challenging enough to stimulate further development, necessitating a change in the training stimulus.

These scientific findings have been instrumental in the development and advocacy of variable resistance training methods. By providing a varying load that adapts to the body's strength curve, variable resistance training can offer more efficient muscle activation, reduce the risk of injury, and help overcome training plateaus. These benefits underscore the importance of considering variable resistance as a potentially more effective and safer alternative to fixed resistance in strength training programs.

# Definition And Science Behind Variable Resistance

Variable Resistance Training (VRT) is a concept in strength and fitness training where the resistance exerted on the muscle changes throughout the range of motion in an exercise. This approach contrasts with traditional weight training, where the resistance remains constant, regardless of the position in the movement. The science behind variable resistance is rooted in the understanding of the body's muscle mechanics and how they respond to different loads.

At the heart of VRT is the concept of the muscle's strength curve, which describes how a muscle's capacity to generate force changes throughout its range of motion. In any given movement, there are points where the muscle is stronger and can handle more load, and points where it is weaker. Traditional weights cannot accommodate this variability – they provide a constant load that doesn't change to match the muscle's changing strength capacity.

Variable resistance aims to align the resistance with the muscle's strength curve more closely. For instance, in a bicep curl, the muscle is weaker at the start and end of the curl but stronger in the middle. VRT would involve using a mechanism, like resistance bands or specially designed weight machines, that increases the load in the middle of the curl and decreases it at the start and end.

This approach ensures that the muscle is optimally challenged throughout the entire movement, leading to more efficient muscle activation and growth.

Another scientific aspect of VRT is its potential to reduce injury risk. By decreasing resistance where the muscle is weakest, VRT reduces the strain on joints and connective tissues at these vulnerable points. This is especially beneficial in exercises where the risk of injury is high due to heavy loads being lifted in mechanically disadvantaged positions.

# Benefits Over Fixed Resistance (Weights)

Variable Resistance Training (VRT) offers several benefits over traditional fixed resistance weight training, primarily due to its adaptability and alignment with the body's natural strength capacities. One of the main advantages is optimized muscle activation. In VRT, the resistance changes in accordance with the muscle's strength curve throughout the range of motion. This means that muscles are challenged more effectively at their strongest points, leading to potentially better muscle growth and strength gains. For instance, in an exercise like the bench press, VRT can increase the resistance in the mid-range, where the muscles are strongest, unlike fixed weights that provide the same resistance throughout.

Another significant benefit is the reduced risk of injury. Fixed weights can place excessive strain on muscles and joints, especially at the weakest points in the range of motion. VRT mitigates this by lowering the resistance where the muscles are less capable of handling heavy loads, such as at the start and end of a bicep curl. This reduction in load at critical points can help prevent joint strain and muscle tears.

VRT also helps in overcoming training plateaus. In traditional weight training, muscles can become accustomed to the constant resistance, leading to a plateau in progress. Variable resistance, by continually changing the load, presents a constantly evolving challenge to the muscles, encouraging continuous growth and improvement.

Moreover, VRT can lead to more balanced muscle development. By providing a varying load, it ensures that all parts of the muscle are adequately stimulated, unlike fixed weights which might only effectively target certain parts of the muscle depending on the exercise.

Finally, VRT can offer more versatility and adaptability in training. It allows for a range of resistance levels within a single exercise, making it suitable for various fitness levels and goals. This adaptability can be particularly beneficial for rehabilitation purposes, where gradually increasing or varying resistance can aid in recovery without the risk of re-injury.

# Overview Of Different Types Of Variable Resistance Equipment

Variable Resistance Training (VRT) utilizes a variety of equipment to modify the resistance throughout an exercise's range of motion. This equipment is designed to align the load with the body's natural strength curve, providing an effective and often safer training experience.

One common type of VRT equipment is resistance bands. These bands come in various sizes and tension levels, offering resistance that increases as they are stretched. This feature makes them ideal for adding variable resistance to exercises like squats, bench presses, or bicep curls. They are particularly popular due to their versatility and portability.

Another type is adjustable resistance machines. These are specialized gym machines designed to change the resistance at different points in an exercise. They often use cams or levers to alter the mechanical advantage, thereby varying the load throughout the movement. These machines are particularly effective for isolating specific muscle groups and are a staple in many gyms.

Chain and band-loaded free weights are also used for VRT. By attaching chains or bands to barbells or dumbbells, the resistance changes with the movement. For example, in a squat, as the lifter stands up and the chains lift off the ground, the resistance increases, matching the body's increasing strength capacity.

Pneumatic resistance equipment, which uses air pressure to provide resistance, is another innovative VRT tool. These machines allow for precise control of the resistance level and can be adjusted quickly and easily, making them suitable for various exercises and fitness levels.

Hydraulic resistance machines are also a form of VRT equipment. They use fluid to create resistance, and the harder or faster the user moves, the more resistance they experience. This type of equipment is often found in rehabilitation centers due to its smooth resistance and low impact on joints.

Lastly, spring resistance equipment, which utilizes springs to create varying resistance, is sometimes used in VRT. The resistance changes depending on how much the spring is stretched or compressed during the exercise.

Each type of variable resistance equipment offers unique benefits and can be used for different training objectives, from muscle building and strength training to rehabilitation and functional fitness. The choice of equipment depends on the specific goals, preferences, and training level of the individual.

# The Body's Natural Strength Curve

Variable Resistance Training (VRT) is highly effective because it complements the body's natural strength curve, a concept crucial to understanding why VRT can be more efficient than traditional fixed resistance training. The natural strength curve refers to the way a muscle's ability to produce force changes throughout its range of motion in any given movement.

In many exercises, muscles are not equally strong at all points of the movement. For example, during a bicep curl, the muscle is weaker at the start and end positions but stronger in the middle. Traditional weights provide a constant load, which means they can be too heavy for the weaker points and too light for the strongest points in the muscle's range of motion. This discrepancy can lead to suboptimal muscle activation and a higher risk of injury.

Variable resistance, on the other hand, adjusts the load to match these variations in muscle strength. This is typically achieved through mechanisms like resistance bands, chains, or specialized weight machines. For instance, resistance bands provide less resistance when they are not stretched much (at the beginning and end of a bicep curl) and more resistance when stretched to a greater extent (at the midpoint of the curl). This changing resistance ensures that the muscle is adequately challenged throughout the entire movement, maximizing muscle activation and growth.

By aligning the resistance with the body's natural strength curve, VRT also reduces the risk of injury. It reduces the load at the points where the muscle and joint are at their weakest and most vulnerable, such as at the bottom of a squat or the start of a shoulder press. This approach minimizes undue stress on joints and connective tissues, making the exercise safer.

Furthermore, VRT's alignment with the strength curve can lead to more balanced muscle development. In fixed resistance training, the inability to lift a weight through the full range of motion (due to weaker points) can result in underdeveloped muscle areas. VRT ensures that all parts of the muscle are worked effectively, leading to more uniform muscle growth.

# Band Only Exercises

These exercises using resistance bands offer a diverse and effective way to target different muscle groups, enhancing strength and stability throughout the body.

Banded Squats are a great way to add resistance to a traditional squat. By standing on the band and holding its ends at shoulder height, you introduce tension throughout the movement. As you squat down, the resistance lessens slightly, aligning with the natural strength curve of your legs. As you stand back up, the tension increases, providing more resistance when your legs are strongest. This added resistance during the ascent phase makes the exercise more challenging and effective for strengthening the lower body muscles.

Banded Push-Ups introduce a new level of challenge to the classic push-up. Placing a band across your back and under your hands adds resistance, particularly at the top of the movement when you push your body up. This extra resistance engages the chest, triceps, and shoulder muscles more intensely than regular push-ups, enhancing muscle activation and strength development in the upper body.

Standing Bicep Curls with a resistance band are an effective way to target the biceps. Standing on the band and performing curls with the arms moving from a fully extended position to bending towards the shoulders creates variable resistance. The tension increases as you curl up, providing more resistance at the point of peak contraction, which can lead to improved muscle engagement and growth in the biceps.

Tricep Band Kickbacks focus on the triceps. By hinging forward at the hips and extending one arm back at a time while holding the band, you create a movement that targets the triceps through a full range of motion. The band's resistance increases as you extend your arm, making the exercise more challenging and effective for tricep development.

Banded Lateral Walks are excellent for targeting the lower body, particularly the glutes and hip abductor muscles. Placing a band around your ankles or thighs and performing side steps maintains constant tension in the band. This continuous resistance during lateral movement helps in strengthening and toning the outer thighs and glutes, which are often neglected in standard lower-body exercises.

Overhead Band Pull Aparts are a great exercise for the shoulders and upper back. By holding the band above your head and stretching it by pulling your arms apart, you engage the deltoid, trapezius, and rhomboid muscles. This exercise is excellent for improving shoulder mobility and strengthening the muscles that support good posture.

Bent Over Rows with a resistance band target the back muscles, including the latissimus dorsi, rhomboids, and lower back. Standing on the band and hinging at the waist, you create a rowing motion that mimics the movement of traditional rowing exercises. The resistance band provides a consistent tension throughout the movement, enhancing muscle engagement and development.

Banded Leg Presses are an innovative way to simulate a leg press exercise without a machine. Lying on your back with the band around your feet and pressing upwards challenges the quadriceps, hamstrings, and glutes. This exercise is beneficial for building lower body strength and can be particularly useful for those who don't have access to leg press equipment.

Front Raises with a resistance band effectively work the anterior deltoids, the front part of the shoulder. Standing on the band and lifting your arms straight in front of you to shoulder height with controlled motion provides resistance that increases with the lift. This exercise is crucial for shoulder development and can help improve shoulder stability.

Banded Glute Bridges focus on the glutes and hips. Lying on your back with a band above your knees, you create tension in the band by keeping your knees apart as you lift your hips. This exercise not only strengthens the glutes but also engages the hip abductors and core muscles, making it a comprehensive lower body workout.

Band Pull-Aparts are excellent for strengthening the muscles in the upper back and shoulders. By holding the band in front of you and pulling it apart, you engage the rear deltoids and the muscles around the shoulder blades, including the rhomboids and trapezius. This exercise is particularly beneficial for counteracting the effects of poor posture and strengthening muscles critical for shoulder health.

The Standing Chest Press with a resistance band is a great alternative to traditional chest press exercises. By anchoring the band behind you and pressing your arms forward, you mimic the movement of a chest press. This exercise targets the pectoral muscles, as well as the triceps and front shoulders. It's a functional exercise that can improve pushing movements in daily activities.

The Shoulder Press with a resistance band is an effective way to strengthen the shoulders and upper arms. Stepping on the band and pressing your hands overhead challenges the entire shoulder region, including the anterior, medial, and posterior deltoids, as well as the triceps. This exercise helps in improving overhead lifting capabilities and shoulder stability.

Banded Planks introduce an additional element of resistance to the traditional plank exercise. With the band around your back and holding the ends with your hands, the exercise becomes more challenging, engaging the core muscles more intensively. This variation not only strengthens the abdominal and lower back muscles but also enhances overall core stability, which is crucial for good posture and balance.

The Single-Leg Banded Hamstring Curl focuses on the hamstrings, one of the key muscle groups in the back of the thigh. By attaching the band to a stable object and your ankle, then curling your leg towards your buttocks, you create targeted resistance for the hamstrings. This exercise is particularly useful for strengthening these muscles, which are crucial for knee stability and injury prevention.

Banded Woodchoppers are an excellent exercise for the core, specifically targeting the obliques, and also engaging the shoulders and hips. By attaching the band to a stable object at shoulder height and pulling it diagonally across the body while twisting the torso, you mimic a chopping motion. This exercise not only strengthens the core muscles but also improves rotational mobility and functional strength, which is beneficial for various sports and daily activities.

Banded Russian Twists are a dynamic way to target the abdominal muscles, particularly the obliques. Sitting on the ground with the band around your feet and twisting your torso while holding the band with both hands adds resistance to the twist motion. This increased resistance enhances the exercise's effectiveness in strengthening the core and improving rotational stability.

Banded Side Bends focus on the obliques and the entire lateral side of the torso. Standing with the band under one foot and holding the other end with the same side hand, you create resistance as you bend sideways. This exercise is key for developing lateral core strength and can help improve side-to-side movements and stability.

Standing Hip Abduction targets the outer thighs and hip abductors. By attaching a band to a stable object and your ankle, and then moving your leg away from your body, you create resistance that challenges these muscles. This exercise is crucial for hip stability and strength, which can benefit overall lower body functionality and balance.

Banded Ankle Jumps add a plyometric element to resistance band training. With a band looped around your ankles and performing small jumps while maintaining tension in the band, you engage the lower leg muscles, including the calves and stabilizers around the ankles. This exercise can enhance lower body power, coordination, and agility, making it particularly beneficial for athletes or those looking to improve explosive movements.

Incorporating these banded exercises into a workout routine can provide varied and effective training, targeting key muscle groups and enhancing overall physical performance. As with all exercises, maintaining proper form and adjusting the resistance to match your fitness level are important to ensure safety and effectiveness.

# Creating Personalized Variable Resistance Programs

Creating personalized variable resistance programs involves careful consideration of an individual's fitness level, goals, and any physical limitations or injuries. The key to a successful program lies in understanding how variable resistance can be effectively integrated to meet these specific needs.

The first step in designing a personalized program is to assess the individual's current fitness level. This includes understanding their strength, endurance, flexibility, and any past injuries or areas of concern. This assessment helps in tailoring the resistance levels and exercises to the individual's capabilities, ensuring safety and effectiveness.

Next, it's important to define clear fitness goals. Whether the aim is to increase muscle strength, improve endurance, enhance flexibility, or rehabilitate from an injury, the program should be aligned with these objectives. For instance, someone looking to build strength might focus on lower repetitions with higher resistance, whereas endurance training would involve higher repetitions with moderate resistance.

Incorporating a variety of exercises is crucial in a variable resistance program. This not only helps in targeting different muscle groups for overall fitness but also prevents monotony and keeps the individual engaged. Exercises should be selected based on how well they suit the individual's goals and physical condition. For example, someone with a knee injury might benefit from low-impact exercises with bands or machines that offer controlled resistance.

The choice of variable resistance equipment is another critical aspect. Options like resistance bands, adjustable resistance machines, and free weights with band or chain attachments can all be effective. The selection should depend on the individual's comfort, the specific muscles being targeted, and the desired outcome of the training.

Progression is a fundamental principle in any training program. Gradually increasing the resistance, changing the exercises, and varying the number of sets and repetitions are essential for continued improvement. This progression should be carefully monitored and adjusted based on the individual's feedback and progress.

Recovery and rest are as important as the workouts themselves. Adequate rest periods should be included in the program to allow muscles to recover and grow. Additionally, incorporating elements like stretching, hydration, and proper nutrition can significantly enhance the program's effectiveness.

Finally, regular reassessment is necessary to track progress and make adjustments to the program as needed. This ensures that the individual continues to progress towards their goals and remains engaged and motivated.

# Consideration Of Different Fitness Levels And Goals

When designing a variable resistance training program, it's essential to consider the diverse fitness levels and goals of individuals. This consideration ensures that the program is effective, safe, and tailored to meet specific needs and aspirations.

For beginners or those with a lower fitness level, the focus should be on building foundational strength and mastering proper form. The program for them should start with lower resistance to minimize the risk of injury and to allow for a focus on technique. Exercises can be simple and involve basic movements that engage major muscle groups. Progression should be gradual, with small increases in resistance as strength and confidence build.

For intermediate-level individuals, the program can introduce more complexity and higher resistance. At this stage, participants are likely to have a good grasp of exercise techniques and can handle more challenging workouts. The program can include a wider range of exercises, targeting specific muscle groups and incorporating a mix of compound and isolation movements. Variable resistance can be used more dynamically at this level, adjusting resistance to match the increased capacity of the muscles.

Advanced individuals usually have specific goals, such as muscle building, strength improvement, endurance enhancement, or athletic performance. Their programs can be highly specialized, with precise manipulation of resistance, volume, and intensity. Advanced techniques, such as supersets, drop sets, or pyramid training, can be incorporated. For these individuals, variable resistance can be maximized to align with their high level of training and specific goals.

In addition to fitness levels, individual goals must also be taken into account. For instance, a program aimed at muscle growth will differ significantly from one designed for weight loss or endurance training. Muscle growth might focus on higher resistance and lower repetitions, while endurance training would involve lower resistance but higher repetitions. Weight loss programs might integrate circuit training with variable resistance to maximize calorie burn.

Regardless of the level or goal, safety should always be a priority. This includes ensuring proper form, using suitable resistance levels, and allowing for adequate rest and recovery. Personalization also means considering any physical limitations or injuries, adapting exercises and resistance to accommodate these constraints.

# Tips For Incorporating Variable Resistance

Integrating variable resistance into existing workout routines can significantly enhance the effectiveness of your training. To do this effectively, it's important to start by incorporating variable resistance elements into exercises that are already familiar. For instance, attaching resistance bands to a barbell during squats or bench presses is a straightforward way to add variable resistance without drastically altering your routine. The integration should be gradual, starting with one or two exercises per workout to allow your body to adapt to the new form of resistance.

When choosing exercises, it's beneficial to balance compound movements with isolation exercises. Variable resistance can greatly augment compound exercises like squats by challenging your muscles more intensively at their strongest points. It's equally effective in isolation movements, such as bicep curls, promoting balanced muscle development. Exploring a variety of variable resistance equipment, like resistance bands or adjustable resistance machines, can add diversity and depth to your workout.

It's also crucial to adjust the volume and intensity of your workouts when incorporating variable resistance. This type of training can be more demanding, so you may need to start with lower reps or sets and increase them gradually. Focus on the engagement of your muscles during exercises; variable resistance can change the feel of an exercise, and being mindful of muscle activation can help you maximize the benefits.

Variable resistance tools are also excellent for warm-ups and cool-downs. They can be used for dynamic stretching to activate muscles before heavier lifting and to aid in recovery post-workout. Experimenting with different resistance levels is key to finding the right challenge for your workouts. Make sure to prioritize safety by checking the condition of bands or equipment and securing them properly to avoid injuries. If you're uncertain about how to effectively integrate variable resistance into your routine, consider seeking advice from a fitness professional. They can offer personalized guidance to ensure your workout plan aligns with your goals and fitness level. Incorporating variable resistance can revitalize your workout routine, offering new challenges and leading to improvements in strength, flexibility, and overall fitness.

Tips and methods:

- Start with Familiar Exercises: Begin by adding variable resistance to exercises you are already comfortable with. This can be as simple as attaching resistance bands to the bar during squats, bench presses, or deadlifts. This approach allows you to focus on adapting to the new resistance pattern without having to learn a new exercise altogether.

- Gradual Integration: Introduce variable resistance gradually. If your routine is predominantly based on fixed weights, start by replacing one or two exercises per workout with their variable resistance counterparts. This gradual shift can help your body adapt without overwhelming it.

- Balance Compound and Isolation Movements: Variable resistance can be particularly effective in compound movements like squats and bench presses, where it can challenge your muscles more at their strongest points. However, it's also beneficial in isolation exercises, like bicep curls or leg extensions, to ensure balanced muscle development.

- Use a Variety of Equipment: Explore different types of variable resistance equipment. Resistance bands are versatile and can be used in a variety of ways, from simple band-only exercises to augmenting free weights. Equipment like adjustable resistance machines or kettlebells with adjustable weights can also offer a variable resistance experience.

- Adjust Volume and Intensity: When incorporating variable resistance, you may need to adjust the volume (reps and sets) and intensity (resistance level) of your workouts. Variable resistance can be more challenging, so you might start with fewer reps or sets and gradually increase as you get used to it.

- Focus on Muscle Engagement: Pay attention to how your muscles engage during the exercise. Variable resistance can alter the feel of an exercise, and focusing on muscle engagement can help you maximize the benefits of the varying resistance levels.

- Incorporate into Warm-Ups and Cool-Downs: Use variable resistance tools like bands for warm-ups and cool-downs. They are excellent for dynamic stretching and activating muscles before heavier lifting, and for helping muscles relax and recover post-workout.

- Experiment with Resistance Levels: Don't be afraid to experiment with different resistance levels. The beauty of variable resistance is its adaptability, so find the resistance bands or settings that challenge you without compromising your form.

- Prioritize Safety: As with any workout routine, safety is paramount. Ensure that any bands or equipment used are in good condition and secured properly to avoid injury.

- Seek Professional Guidance if Needed: If you're unsure about how to integrate variable resistance effectively into your routine, consider consulting a fitness professional. They can provide personalized advice and ensure your workout plan aligns with your goals and fitness level.

## Comparative Analysis With Weight Training Outcomes

When comparing the outcomes of Variable Resistance Training (VRT) with traditional weight training, it's important to consider various factors including muscle development, strength gains, risk of injury, and overall fitness improvements. Each method has distinct characteristics that influence these outcomes.

Variable Resistance Training is designed to align closely with the body's natural strength curves. This means that the resistance changes in accordance with the muscle's ability to produce force at different points in an exercise. As a result, VRT can lead to more comprehensive muscle activation throughout the entire range of motion. This potentially leads to more balanced and efficient muscle development, as muscles are adequately challenged at both their strongest and weakest points. Furthermore, VRT often results in a lower risk of injury. The varying resistance decreases the load at points where the muscles and joints are most vulnerable, reducing the likelihood of strain and overuse injuries.

Traditional weight training, on the other hand, offers constant resistance. This consistency can be beneficial for building raw strength and muscle mass, as it allows for straightforward progression in lifting heavier weights. However, because the resistance does not change, it might not target muscle fibers as effectively throughout the entire range of motion. There's a higher risk of injury with traditional weights, particularly if lifting heavy, due to the constant load on muscles and joints. Overuse injuries and issues related to muscle imbalances are also more common in traditional weight training, especially if there's a lack of variety in the exercises.

In terms of strength gains, both VRT and traditional weight training can be effective, but they may excel in different areas. Traditional weight training is often seen as superior for maximal strength development, given its focus on lifting heavier loads. VRT, while also effective for building strength, might offer greater benefits in terms of functional strength and endurance, as it trains muscles across a wider range of motion and varying levels of resistance.

For overall fitness, VRT provides a more dynamic workout that can adapt to different fitness levels and goals. It's particularly beneficial for those who require a training regime that accommodates for fluctuating strength levels, such as individuals in rehabilitation or those with specific sports performance goals.

In conclusion, both Variable Resistance Training and traditional weight training have their unique advantages. The choice between them should be based on individual goals, fitness levels, and preferences. VRT offers more comprehensive muscle development, lower injury risk, and functional strength, while traditional weight training is excellent for building maximal strength and muscle mass. Combining elements of both methods could provide a comprehensive approach to strength and fitness training.

## Free Weights Combined With Bands

Combining the stability and feedback of free weights with the progressive resistance of bands creates a hybrid training method that leverages the benefits of both systems. This approach can offer a more comprehensive and effective strength training experience.

Free weights, such as barbells and dumbbells, are revered for their ability to provide stability and feedback. They engage not only the primary muscle groups targeted by specific exercises but also the stabilizing muscles. This engagement is crucial for building functional strength and enhancing proprioception, the body's ability to sense its position and movement. Free weights also offer straightforward feedback in terms of weight lifted, allowing for clear measurement of strength gains.

Resistance bands, on the other hand, offer progressive resistance. This means that the resistance increases as the band stretches, aligning more closely with the body's natural strength curve. As a muscle extends through its range of motion, it generally becomes stronger, and resistance bands match this increase in strength. This quality of bands helps in providing a more consistent and evenly distributed muscle activation throughout the entire range of motion of an exercise.

To combine these two methods, resistance bands can be used in conjunction with free weights. For example, in a bench press, bands can be anchored to the bench or the floor and attached to the barbell. As the barbell is pressed upwards, the bands stretch, increasing the resistance. This setup maintains the stability and feedback of the barbell while adding a variable resistance component that challenges the muscles more as they reach their strongest point.

Similarly, in exercises like squats or deadlifts, bands can be attached to the barbell and an anchor point on the ground. As the lifter ascends in a squat or lifts in a deadlift, the resistance from the bands increases, providing a greater challenge at the top of the movement where the lifter is typically strongest.

This combination not only enhances muscle activation throughout the range of motion but also adds an element of dynamic resistance, making the muscles work harder at their peak capacity. It can lead to improved muscle growth, greater strength gains, and potentially a reduced risk of injury, as the variable resistance from the bands can ease the load on the muscles and joints at their weakest points.

## Equipment Setup

Setting up equipment for a hybrid training program that combines free weights and resistance bands requires a careful arrangement to ensure safety and effectiveness. The primary components of this setup include free weights, resistance bands, and a secure anchoring system.

Free weights form the foundation of this setup. Standard barbells, dumbbells, or kettlebells are used depending on the exercise. These weights are chosen for their ability to provide a stable and predictable load, which is essential for muscle development and strength training. The selection of free weights depends on the user's strength level and the specific exercises planned in the workout routine.

Resistance bands are the second crucial element. A variety of bands with different tension levels are necessary to accommodate various exercises and strength levels. These bands can offer progressive resistance, increasing the difficulty of an exercise as they stretch. Having a range of bands allows for a more tailored workout where the resistance can be adjusted according to the specific needs of the exercise and the individual's capabilities.

The anchoring system is a critical component to ensure safety and functionality. The bands need to be securely anchored to provide consistent resistance and prevent snapping back, which could lead to injury. Anchoring points can be on the ground, on a squat rack, or any other stable structure that can safely bear the tension of the bands. For ground anchoring, heavy-duty hooks or anchors that can be attached to the floor are used. If a squat rack or similar structure is used, the bands should be securely fastened to the rack in a manner that doesn't impede the movement of the free weights but still provides the necessary tension.

This setup provides the versatility needed for a range of exercises. For example, in a squat or a deadlift, bands can be anchored to the ground and attached to either end of a barbell, increasing resistance as the lifter stands up. For exercises like bench presses or shoulder presses, bands can be anchored to the bench or the ground and attached to the barbell, adding resistance as the bar is pushed away from the body.

# Safety and Preparation

Safety and preparation are paramount in any workout routine, especially when combining free weights with resistance bands. Proper warm-up, safety checks, and appropriate progression are critical components to ensure a safe and effective workout.

A thorough warm-up is essential to prepare the muscles and joints for the workout. Warming up increases blood flow to the muscles, enhances flexibility, and reduces the risk of injury. A good warm-up should include dynamic stretches and light aerobic exercises to activate the muscles that will be used in the workout. Activities like jogging in place, arm circles, leg swings, and light exercises using lower resistance bands can be particularly effective. This preparatory phase helps to gradually raise the heart rate and prepare the body for the more strenuous activity to follow.

Safety checks of all equipment before starting the workout are crucial. This involves ensuring that the free weights, such as barbells and dumbbells, are in good condition and that the weight plates (if used) are securely fastened. For resistance bands, it's vital to check for any signs of wear or damage, such as small tears or fraying, which could lead to the band snapping during use. The anchoring system for the bands must be thoroughly inspected to ensure that it is secure and can withstand the tension of the bands during exercises. This includes checking that the bands are correctly attached to the anchor points and that these points are stable and immovable.

Starting with lighter weights and lower tension bands is advisable, especially for those who are new to this type of training or for the first few exercises in a session. Beginning with lighter resistance allows the body to adapt to the combined demands of free weights and bands. It also provides an opportunity to focus on proper form and technique, which is crucial for preventing injuries. As the muscles warm up and adapt to the exercise routine, the resistance can be progressively increased. This gradual progression helps to ensure that the body is not overwhelmed, reducing the risk of strain or injury.

## Key Compound Movements

The methodology for incorporating variable resistance into key compound movements, specifically the squat, involves a strategic setup and execution to enhance the effectiveness of the exercise. The squat, being a fundamental compound movement, benefits significantly from the addition of variable resistance, as it can better match the body's natural strength curve.

# Squat

Setup for Squat with Variable Resistance:

- Attaching Bands: Begin by securely attaching resistance bands to the bottom of the squat rack. The bands should be placed such that they can extend to the ends of the barbell. Ensure that the bands are of equal length and tension on both sides to maintain balance during the squat.

- Positioning the Barbell: Load the barbell with the desired weight as you would for a regular squat. Then, carefully attach each end of the barbell to the resistance bands. It's important to check that the bands are securely fastened to the barbell and that they provide a uniform resistance when stretched.

- Safety Check: Before starting the exercise, perform a safety check to ensure that the bands are correctly attached and that the squat rack is stable. This check is crucial to prevent any accidents during the workout.

Execution of Squat with Variable Resistance:

- Starting Position: Position yourself under the barbell, placing it across your shoulders as you would for a conventional squat. Keep your feet shoulder-width apart, and ensure your grip on the bar is balanced.

- Performing the Squat: Begin the squat by bending your knees and lowering your body as if sitting back into a chair. Keep your back straight, and your core engaged throughout the movement.

- Ascending with Resistance: As you ascend back to the standing position, the resistance bands will stretch, increasing the resistance. This increase in resistance aligns with the point in the squat where your legs are strongest, thereby providing a more effective muscle engagement.

- Completing the Repetition: Continue to stand up until your legs are nearly straight, then lower back down into the next squat, maintaining control and proper form throughout the movement.

By using resistance bands in conjunction with free weights in the squat, you add a progressive resistance element to the exercise. This method enhances muscle activation, particularly in the upward phase of the squat, and aligns the resistance with the body's increasing strength as you stand up. The result is a more dynamic and challenging squat that can lead to improved strength and muscle development compared to traditional squats with fixed resistance.

# Bench Press

Incorporating variable resistance into the bench press exercise involves a setup where resistance bands are used in conjunction with the barbell. This setup aims to increase the resistance during the upward phase of the press, which can enhance muscle activation and overall strength, particularly at the lockout phase of the lift.

Setup for Bench Press with Variable Resistance:

- Securing Bands: The first step is to secure the resistance bands beneath the bench or to a stable ground anchor point located near the head of the bench. The bands should be positioned so that they can be attached to each end of the barbell. It's essential to ensure that the bands are of equal length and tension on both sides for balanced resistance.

- Attaching Bands to Barbell: Once the bands are securely in place, attach each end of the barbell to the bands. Carefully load the barbell with the desired weight, keeping in mind that the bands will add additional resistance during the lift.

- Safety Check: Conduct a thorough safety check to confirm that the bands are securely attached to the barbell and that they won't slip or come loose during the exercise. Also, ensure that the bench is stable and positioned correctly relative to the anchor points of the bands.

Execution of Bench Press with Variable Resistance:

- Starting Position: Lie back on the bench and grip the barbell with your hands slightly wider than shoulder-width apart. Keep your feet flat on the floor and your back flat against the bench.

- Lowering the Bar: Lower the barbell slowly towards your chest, keeping your wrists straight and elbows slightly tucked in. The resistance from the bands will decrease as you lower the bar, allowing you to focus on control and form.

- Pressing Up with Increased Resistance: Push the barbell upwards, extending your arms fully. As you press up, the bands will stretch, increasing the resistance. This added resistance towards the end of the press is particularly effective in strengthening the lockout portion of the bench press.

- Completing the Repetition: Continue pushing until your arms are fully extended, then lower the barbell back down for the next repetition, maintaining a smooth and controlled movement throughout.

By using resistance bands in the bench press, the exercise becomes more challenging at the point where the arms are strongest, which is typically towards the end of the press. This setup can lead to increased strength, particularly in the triceps and chest muscles, as they are required to work harder against the increased resistance during the lockout. It also adds a dynamic aspect to the bench press, potentially leading to greater muscle growth and strength gains compared to using a fixed resistance alone.

## Deadlift

Incorporating variable resistance into the deadlift involves a setup where resistance bands are anchored to a solid base and attached to the barbell. This method enhances the exercise by increasing the resistance during the lifting phase, which can simulate a heavier weight as the lifter reaches full extension, thereby intensifying the workout, especially in the latter part of the lift where the body is typically stronger.

Setup for Deadlift with Variable Resistance:

- Anchoring Bands: Start by anchoring the resistance bands to a solid and stable base on the ground. This base could be heavy-duty hooks or anchor points specifically designed for band attachment. It's important that the anchor point is directly below where the barbell will be lifted, ensuring a vertical line of resistance.

- Attaching Bands to Barbell: Once the bands are anchored, attach each end of the bands to the barbell, placed on the ground as you would in a regular deadlift setup. Ensure that the bands are evenly attached and provide balanced resistance on both sides of the barbell.

- Safety Check: Before beginning the exercise, perform a safety check to ensure that the bands are securely fastened to the barbell and the anchor point. The bands should be strong enough to withstand the tension of the lift without risk of snapping.

Execution of Deadlift with Variable Resistance:

- Starting Position: Stand with your feet hip-width apart, centering them under the barbell. Bend at the hips and knees to reach down and grasp the barbell with a grip that is shoulder-width apart.

- Initiating the Lift: Begin the deadlift by lifting the barbell off the ground, pushing through your heels and keeping your back straight. As you start lifting, the resistance from the bands will be relatively low.

- Increasing Resistance: As you continue to lift and straighten your body, the resistance from the bands will increase. This increased resistance adds an additional challenge to the lift, particularly as you approach full extension. The bands simulate a heavier weight at the top of the lift, engaging the muscles more intensely.

- Completing the Lift: Fully extend your hips and knees to stand up straight at the top of the lift. The added resistance from the bands at this point maximizes muscle activation. Lower the barbell back to the ground in a controlled manner, ready for the next repetition.

The addition of variable resistance in the deadlift targets the muscles more effectively as they reach their strongest point at full extension. This method not only enhances muscle activation but also adds a new dimension to the exercise, potentially leading to greater strength gains and muscle development, particularly in the glutes, hamstrings, and lower back. It's an effective way to intensify the deadlift while aligning the resistance with the body's natural strength curve.

## Shoulder Press

Setup for Shoulder Press with Variable Resistance:

- Anchoring Bands: Begin by anchoring the resistance bands to a low point. This could be a heavy-duty hook or anchor on the floor or a low part of a squat rack. Ensure that the anchor point is stable and can withstand the tension of the bands during the exercise.

- Attaching Bands to Barbell or Dumbbells: Once the bands are anchored, attach the other end of each band to the barbell or dumbbells. If using a barbell, make sure the bands are attached evenly on both sides to maintain balance. For dumbbells, each dumbbell should have its own band attached.

- Safety Check: Conduct a thorough safety check to ensure that the bands are securely fastened to both the anchor point and the weights. It's crucial that the bands are not stretched to their maximum capacity at the starting position to avoid excessive tension or risk of snapping.

Execution of Shoulder Press with Variable Resistance:

- Starting Position: Sit or stand, depending on your preference for the shoulder press, holding the barbell or dumbbells at shoulder height. Your hands should be positioned just wider than shoulder-width apart for a barbell, and for dumbbells, they should be at the shoulders with palms facing forward.

- Performing the Press: Begin the press by pushing the barbell or dumbbells upwards. As you lift the weights, the resistance bands will stretch, increasing the resistance progressively. This variable resistance challenges the shoulder muscles more as they become stronger during the lift.

- Maximizing Resistance at the Top: Continue pressing until your arms are fully extended above your head. At this top point of the movement, the bands provide maximum resistance, intensifying the workout and maximizing muscle engagement, particularly in the deltoids and triceps.

- Lowering the Weights: Slowly lower the weights back to the starting position at shoulder height, controlling the movement against the tension of the bands. The decreasing resistance helps in managing the weights safely back to the starting position.

This method of performing the shoulder press with variable resistance is highly effective for developing shoulder strength and muscle size. The increasing resistance with the lift's progression allows for a more intense workout at the points where the muscles are strongest, leading to potentially greater gains in strength and muscle development compared to traditional shoulder press exercises.

# Rows

Setup for Rows with Variable Resistance:

- Attaching Bands to a Stable Point: Start by attaching one end of the resistance bands to a stable point in front of where you'll be performing the rows. This could be a heavy-duty hook, a part of a squat rack, or any other secure anchor point at about waist height. The anchor should be able to hold the tension of the bands during the rowing motion.

- Extending Bands to Barbell or Dumbbells: Once the bands are anchored, extend them and attach the other end to the barbell or dumbbells. If using a barbell, ensure that the bands are attached evenly on both sides. For dumbbells, attach a band to each dumbbell.

- Safety Check: Conduct a comprehensive safety check to make sure that the bands are securely attached at both ends and that they are not overly stretched in the starting position. This step is crucial to prevent the bands from snapping or coming loose during the exercise.

Execution of Rows with Variable Resistance:

- Starting Position: Stand (or sit, if doing seated rows) facing the anchor point, holding the barbell or dumbbells with your hands. Your feet should be shoulder-width apart for stability, and your knees slightly bent.

- Performing the Row: Begin the row by pulling the weights towards your body. Keep your back straight and engage your core throughout the movement. As you pull, the resistance bands will stretch, increasing the tension as you move through the row.

- Stronger Peak Contraction: Continue pulling the weights towards your lower abdomen or chest, depending on the type of row. As the bands stretch further, they provide increased resistance, leading to a stronger peak contraction in the back muscles. This added resistance at the point of peak contraction enhances the effectiveness of the exercise, particularly targeting the mid and upper back muscles.

- Returning to Starting Position: After reaching the peak contraction, slowly release the weights back to the starting position, controlling the movement against the tension of the bands. This controlled release helps maintain muscle engagement throughout the entire range of motion.

Adding variable resistance to rows can significantly improve muscle activation and development in the back, offering a more challenging and effective workout compared to traditional rowing exercises. The increased resistance at the point of peak contraction enhances the exercise's intensity, potentially leading to better strength gains and muscle growth.

## Programming Considerations

When incorporating variable resistance into a workout program, it's crucial to consider programming elements such as volume, intensity, progressive overload, and variation. These factors play a significant role in ensuring the effectiveness of the training while minimizing the risk of injury.

Volume and intensity are key components of any workout program. When combining free weights with resistance bands, it's important to find the right balance between the weight of the free weights and the tension of the bands. This combination should be adjusted to suit the individual's fitness level and training goals. For instance, a focus on strength building might require lower repetitions with higher intensity, meaning heavier weights and bands with greater resistance. Conversely, a focus on endurance or muscle toning might call for higher repetitions with moderate intensity.

Progressive overload is a fundamental principle in strength training and fitness. It involves gradually increasing the resistance or load to continuously challenge the muscles, leading to improved strength and muscle development. In a variable resistance program, this can be achieved by either increasing the weights, using bands with higher tension, or a combination of both. It's important to increase the resistance progressively to ensure consistent muscle growth and strength gains while avoiding overtraining or injury.

Variation in the workout routine is another crucial aspect. Regularly changing the band tension and the weight can help to challenge the muscles in different ways, preventing adaptation and plateauing. This variation can be in the form of altering the exercises, adjusting the resistance, modifying the number of sets and repetitions, or changing the tempo of the exercises. Incorporating different types of variable resistance equipment can also add diversity to the workouts, further challenging the muscles and making the training more interesting and engaging.

## Monitoring and Adjustment

Monitoring and adjustment are critical aspects of any workout program, especially when incorporating variable resistance. These processes involve paying close attention to body feedback and making necessary adjustments to the training regimen to optimize effectiveness and prevent injury.

Body feedback is an invaluable source of information. It involves being attentive to how the body responds during and after workouts. This includes monitoring muscle soreness, joint discomfort, fatigue levels, and overall performance. If there is excessive soreness or joint pain, it might indicate that the joints are being overloaded, or the workout intensity is too high. In such cases, it's crucial to scale back the resistance or modify the exercises to reduce the strain on the body. Listening to your body is essential to avoid overtraining and injuries, which can set back progress significantly.

Adjustment of the training variables is a key response to the feedback received. If a workout feels too challenging or is causing discomfort, reducing the band tension or the weight can help. Similarly, if the exercises feel too easy or if there's no noticeable progression, it may be time to increase the resistance. These adjustments should be made thoughtfully, considering both performance and comfort.

Regular adjustment is not only a response to feedback but also a proactive measure to continually challenge the muscles. As the body adapts to a certain level of resistance, it becomes important to modify the training variables to ensure ongoing improvement. This can be done by increasing the weight, changing the band tension, varying the exercises, or adjusting other aspects like the number of repetitions or sets.

# Post-Workout Care

Recovery and maintenance are essential components of a comprehensive workout program, particularly one that involves variable resistance training. Effective post-workout care and regular equipment checks are crucial for ensuring ongoing progress and safety.

Post-workout care primarily focuses on strategies that facilitate recovery and reduce the risk of injury. Stretching after a workout is vital for maintaining and improving flexibility, which can enhance overall performance and reduce muscle soreness. Stretching helps in elongating the muscles that have been contracted during the workout, aiding in recovery and reducing the likelihood of muscle tightness and stiffness.

Hydration is another critical aspect of recovery. During a workout, the body loses fluids through sweat, and it's important to replenish these fluids to aid in muscle recovery and prevent dehydration. Proper hydration supports metabolic processes and nutrient transfer within the body, both of which are essential for muscle repair and growth.

Nutrition also plays a significant role in post-workout recovery. Consuming a balanced meal or snack that includes a mix of proteins, carbohydrates, and fats after a workout can help in repairing and building muscle tissues. Proteins are particularly important as they provide the amino acids needed for muscle repair. Carbohydrates help in replenishing glycogen stores that are depleted during exercise.

Regular checks of the workout equipment are equally important to ensure safety and effectiveness. This includes inspecting resistance bands for any signs of wear, tear, or fraying. Given that bands are under constant tension and stress, they can become worn over time, and using damaged bands can lead to injury. Checking the condition of free weights, such as barbells and dumbbells, is also necessary. This involves ensuring that the weights are secure and that there is no damage to the equipment that could pose a safety risk.

## Nutrition: Fueling Your Journey

In the world of bodybuilding, nutrition is your ultimate weapon, your silent partner in the quest for muscle and strength. As you sweat it out in the gym, pushing your limits with every rep, your muscles are screaming for nourishment, and it's your job to feed them. This chapter lays down the foundation of what it means to be a bodybuilder, and how nutrition is the very essence of your journey.

Bodybuilding isn't a mere hobby; it's a lifestyle, a relentless pursuit of physical excellence. To understand its core, we must first delve into its history. Bodybuilding, as we know it today, wasn't born yesterday. It has a rich and gritty history that traces its roots back to ancient Greece, where Herculean physiques were celebrated. But it was in the late 19th century when the sport began to take its modern form. It became a spectacle, with men and women flexing their sculpted bodies, showcasing strength, symmetry, and aesthetics. It wasn't just about being strong; it was about looking strong.

Fast forward to the present day, and bodybuilding has evolved into a multifaceted discipline. It's not just about bulging muscles and flashy poses; it's about sculpting your physique, pushing the limits of your body, and achieving the perfect blend of muscle and symmetry. It's a journey of dedication, discipline, and above all, nutrition.

You see, bodybuilding isn't a sprint; it's a marathon. And in this marathon, nutrition is your fuel. It's what powers your muscles to grow and recover. Without proper nutrition, your bodybuilding dreams are nothing but a house of cards waiting to collapse. You can lift all the weights in the world, but if you don't feed your body right, you'll never reach your true potential.

Now, let's get to the heart of the matter – the importance of nutrition in natural bodybuilding. It's not just about eating; it's about eating with a purpose. You're not shoving food down your throat; you're strategically fueling your body to achieve specific goals. Nutrition in bodybuilding isn't a one-size-fits-all concept. It's tailored to your unique needs, your body type, and your goals.

At the core of bodybuilding nutrition are macronutrients – protein, carbohydrates, and fats. These are the building blocks of your diet, and they play distinct roles in your bodybuilding journey.

Protein, the undisputed champion of macronutrients, is your muscle's best friend. It's the raw material your body needs to repair and grow muscle tissue. Every rep you do in the gym creates tiny tears in your muscle fibers. It's in the post-workout recovery phase that your muscles rebuild themselves, stronger and more massive than before. But they need protein to do so.

Sources of high-quality protein are your go-to weapons. Lean meats like chicken, turkey, and fish, along with dairy products like Greek yogurt and cottage cheese, should be your daily allies. Vegetarians can rely on sources like tofu, lentils, and quinoa to get their protein fix. But remember, it's not just about the quantity of protein; it's about the quality. Protein is your ammunition, so don't settle for anything less than the best.

Carbohydrates, often misunderstood and vilified, are the energy source that keeps your body firing on all cylinders. You've probably heard about low-carb diets and keto crazes, but in the world of bodybuilding, carbs are your friends. They provide the energy you need to fuel your workouts and recover afterward. Carbs are like the gasoline that powers a high-performance engine.

But not all carbs are created equal. Simple carbs, like those found in sugary snacks and sodas, will leave you crashing and burning. Complex carbs, on the other hand, are your secret weapon. Foods like brown rice, oats, sweet potatoes, and whole-grain bread provide a slow and steady release of energy, keeping you pumped throughout your grueling workouts.

Fats, often demonized in the dieting world, are essential for bodybuilders. They are the building blocks of hormones, including testosterone, which plays a critical role in muscle growth. But not all fats are created equal. Healthy fats, found in avocados, nuts, seeds, and fatty fish like salmon, are your allies in the quest for muscle. They also aid in the absorption of fat-soluble vitamins, ensuring your body gets the full nutritional benefit.

It's not about avoiding fats; it's about choosing the right ones. So, when someone tells you to go low-fat, you know better. Embrace the fats that fuel your body and enhance your muscle-building potential.

Now that you understand the role of macronutrients, it's time to put them into action. You're not just eating food; you're crafting a well-thought-out meal plan. The goal is to create a diet that provides the right balance of these macronutrients to support your bodybuilding objectives.

Balancing your macronutrients requires calculating your daily caloric needs. This isn't rocket science, but it does require some effort. You can't just eyeball your food and hope for the best. You need to know how many calories your body needs to maintain its current weight, and from there, you can adjust to achieve your goals.

There are various formulas and online calculators available to estimate your daily calorie needs. Once you have that number, you can determine how many of those calories should come from each macronutrient. For instance, a typical bodybuilding diet might consist of 40% carbohydrates, 30% protein, and 30% fats. This breakdown can be adjusted based on your specific goals.

Creating a meal plan based on these percentages can seem daunting, but it's crucial for success. It's like mapping out your battle strategy before entering the gym. With a well-structured plan, you'll have a clear path to your bodybuilding goals.

Timing is another crucial aspect of natural bodybuilding nutrition. You can't just eat haphazardly and expect results. Pre-workout nutrition sets the stage for your performance. You need a meal or snack that provides a good balance of carbohydrates and protein to fuel your workout and help you push through those heavy sets.

Post-workout nutrition is equally critical. After your intense training session, your muscles are starving for nutrients. This is the time to replenish your glycogen stores with carbohydrates and provide your muscles with the protein they need for recovery and growth. A post-workout shake or a well-balanced meal is your best bet.

Timing isn't just about the pre and post-workout periods; it's about consistency throughout the day. You should aim to eat every 3-4 hours to keep a steady flow of nutrients to your muscles. Skipping meals or going too long without eating can lead to muscle breakdown, the last thing you want as a bodybuilder.

# Macronutrients for Muscle Growth

In the relentless world of bodybuilding, where iron meets sweat and determination collides with the weights, nutrition isn't just a part of the puzzle – it's the bedrock on which your success is built. This chapter, "Macronutrients for Muscle Growth," is all about the raw materials that fuel your body's transformation into a powerhouse of muscle and strength. In this no-nonsense guide, we'll dive straight into the core of bodybuilding nutrition, starting with the heavyweight champion of them all: protein.

Protein: The Cornerstone of Muscle Growth

Protein isn't just another nutrient; it's your ticket to muscle city. When you're pumping iron and pushing your body to the limits, you're essentially tearing down muscle fibers. It's in the recovery phase that your muscles rebuild and grow, and they need protein to do it.

Picture this: every rep, every set, and every drop of sweat are investments in your body's future. But without enough protein, those investments won't yield the returns you crave. Protein is the contractor that repairs the damaged muscle tissue, making it thicker, denser, and more powerful than before.

So, what's the deal with protein sources? Well, think of them as different tools in your muscle-building toolbox. Some are tried-and-true classics, while others are versatile newcomers.

- The Classics: Lean meats like chicken, turkey, and beef are your timeless protein allies. They're packed with essential amino acids, the building blocks of muscle. When you're looking to pack on mass, these should be your first choices. They're lean, mean, and muscle-building machines.

- Dairy Delights: Greek yogurt, cottage cheese, and milk are dairy powerhouses that are rich in protein. They also provide valuable calcium and other nutrients. If you're looking for a creamy way to fuel your muscles, these options are worth considering.

- Plant-Based Players: Not a fan of meat or dairy? No problem. Plant-based protein sources like tofu, lentils, chickpeas, and quinoa can be your go-to options. They offer protein with a side of fiber and an array of essential nutrients.

- Protein Powders: In the fast-paced world of natural bodybuilding, convenience matters. Protein powders, whether whey, casein, or plant-based, are quick and easy sources of protein. They're ideal for post-workout recovery when your muscles are hungry for nutrients.

But here's the deal-breaker – it's not just about the quantity of protein; it's also about the quality. Protein sources vary in terms of amino acid profiles and absorption rates. You want protein sources that are rich in essential amino acids and are easily digestible, ensuring your muscles get the most bang for their buck.

Now, let's talk numbers. How much protein do you need to feed those hungry muscles? The answer depends on various factors, including your body weight, age, activity level, and your specific bodybuilding goals.

For most bodybuilders, a good rule of thumb is to aim for around 1.2 to 2.2 grams of protein per kilogram of body weight daily. This range allows room for customization based on your unique needs. If you're looking to bulk up and pack on muscle, you may lean towards the higher end of the spectrum. If you're in a cutting phase and aiming to shed fat while preserving muscle, the lower end may suffice.

Carbohydrates: The Energy Source

Carbs often get a bad rap in the dieting world, but in the realm of bodybuilding, they're your secret weapon. Carbohydrates are your primary source of energy, the fuel that powers your workouts and recovery.

Picture your body as a high-performance car. It needs the right fuel to perform at its best. Complex carbohydrates are your premium octane. They provide a slow and steady release of energy, keeping you revved up throughout your grueling workouts.

But not all carbs are created equal. You've probably heard of simple carbs and complex carbs. Let's break it down.

- Simple Carbs: These are the sugary, quick-burning carbs found in candy, soda, and other processed junk. They might give you a temporary spike in energy, but they'll leave you crashing and burning soon after.

- Complex Carbs: These are your allies in the quest for muscle. Foods like brown rice, oats, sweet potatoes, whole-grain bread, and legumes provide a sustained release of energy. They keep you going strong, powering through set after set.

Now, here's the kicker – timing matters. Pre-workout nutrition is your opportunity to prime your body for a killer session at the gym. You want a meal or snack that provides a good balance of carbohydrates to fuel your workout and protein to kickstart muscle recovery. Think of it as loading up your car with premium fuel before a race.

Post-workout nutrition is equally crucial. After your intense training session, your muscles are starving for nutrients. This is the time to replenish your glycogen stores with carbohydrates and provide your muscles with the protein they need for recovery and growth. A post-workout shake or a well-balanced meal is your best bet.

But remember, carbohydrates aren't a license to gorge on pizza and pasta. The key is to choose complex carbs that are nutrient-dense and support your bodybuilding goals. You're not just fueling up; you're investing in your body's performance and progress.

- Fats: Essential for Hormone Production

- Fats have long been misunderstood and unfairly demonized in the world of nutrition. But in the world of bodybuilding, they're essential for hormone production, including testosterone, which plays a pivotal role in muscle growth.

- Think of fats as the oil that keeps the gears of your body's engine running smoothly. They're involved in various processes, including nutrient absorption, cell membrane health, and the production of vital hormones. Without enough healthy fats, your bodybuilding journey can hit a roadblock.

- But not all fats are created equal. There are the good guys – healthy fats – and the bad guys – trans fats and excessive saturated fats. Let's focus on the heroes of the story.

- Omega-3 Fatty Acids: Found in fatty fish like salmon, mackerel, and sardines, as well as walnuts and flaxseeds, omega-3 fatty acids are anti-inflammatory powerhouses. They support joint health, reduce muscle soreness, and aid in recovery.

- Monounsaturated Fats: Olive oil, avocados, and nuts are rich in monounsaturated fats. They promote heart health and provide a source of sustainable energy.

- Polyunsaturated Fats: These fats, found in sources like sunflower seeds, soybean oil, and fatty fish, are essential for overall health. They're also involved in maintaining the integrity of cell membranes.

Healthy fats not only keep your body's engine running but also aid in the absorption of fat-soluble vitamins like

A, D, E, and K. So, when you're crafting your bodybuilding diet, don't skimp on fats; choose wisely.

# Micronutrients and Supplements

In the unrelenting world of bodybuilding, where every lift, every repetition, and every drop of sweat counts, micronutrients and supplements are the secret arsenal that can elevate your journey to unprecedented heights. This chapter, "Micronutrients and Supplements," is not about the mainstream hype or miracle pills; it's about the nitty-gritty essentials that can make or break your pursuit of the ultimate physique.

Vitamins and Minerals for Muscle Health

Let's kick things off with the unsung heroes of nutrition – vitamins and minerals. Often overlooked in favor of macronutrients, these micronutrients are the foundation of your body's intricate machinery. They're the nuts and bolts that keep everything running smoothly.

- Vitamin A: Essential for maintaining healthy skin and mucous membranes, vitamin A also supports vision and immune function. It's found in foods like sweet potatoes, carrots, and spinach.

- Vitamin D: Known as the sunshine vitamin, vitamin D plays a crucial role in calcium absorption, bone health, and immune function.

Get your fix from sunlight or fortified foods like fatty fish and fortified dairy products.

- Vitamin C: This antioxidant powerhouse supports collagen production, aids in wound healing, and boosts the immune system. Citrus fruits, strawberries, and bell peppers are excellent sources.

- Vitamin E: With its antioxidant properties, vitamin E helps protect cells from oxidative damage. Nuts, seeds, and vegetable oils are rich sources.

- Vitamin K: Vital for blood clotting and bone metabolism, vitamin K is found in leafy greens like kale, spinach, and broccoli.

- B Vitamins: This group includes B1 (thiamine), B2 (riboflavin), B3 (niacin), B5 (pantothenic acid), B6 (pyridoxine), B7 (biotin), B9 (folate), and B12 (cobalamin). They're involved in energy metabolism, red blood cell formation, and various cellular processes. Whole grains, meat, dairy, and leafy greens are good sources.

- Calcium: Essential for strong bones and muscle function, calcium can be found in dairy products, leafy greens, and fortified foods.

- Iron: Crucial for oxygen transport in the blood and muscle function, iron is abundant in red meat, poultry, fish, and legumes.

- Magnesium: This mineral is involved in muscle contraction and relaxation, energy production, and bone health. You can find it in nuts, seeds, whole grains, and leafy greens.

- Zinc: Essential for immune function and protein synthesis, zinc is prevalent in meat, dairy, nuts, and legumes.

- Selenium: An antioxidant that supports thyroid function and immune health, selenium is found in nuts, seeds, and seafood.

- Potassium: Crucial for muscle contractions and nerve impulses, potassium is abundant in bananas, potatoes, and citrus fruits.

These micronutrients aren't just fancy buzzwords. They're the vitamins and minerals your body needs to operate at peak performance. They're not optional; they're mandatory for the meticulous process of sculpting muscle and achieving your bodybuilding goals. Deficiencies can derail your progress faster than you can say "biceps."

The Role of Supplements

Now, let's talk about supplements – those pills, powders, and potions that promise to take your gains to the next level. Supplements can be a valuable addition to your bodybuilding toolkit, but they're not magic bullets. It's crucial to understand their role and use them wisely.

- Pre-Workout Supplements: These are designed to boost energy, focus, and endurance before hitting the gym. They often contain caffeine, creatine, and amino acids. While they can provide a temporary performance boost, they're not a substitute for a solid nutrition plan and should be used in moderation.

- Protein Supplements: Protein shakes and powders are convenient sources of protein, especially post-workout when your muscles need it the most. They're not a replacement for whole-food sources of protein but can be a useful tool for meeting your daily protein intake goals.

- Recovery Supplements: Branched-Chain Amino Acids (BCAAs) and glutamine are often marketed as recovery aids. While there's some evidence to suggest they may reduce muscle soreness and support recovery, they should complement a well-rounded diet rather than replace it.

- Vitamins and Minerals: If you have specific micronutrient deficiencies or struggle to meet your daily requirements through food alone, multivitamin and mineral supplements can be a safety net. However, it's best to get your nutrients from whole foods whenever possible.

- Fish Oil: Omega-3 fatty acids, found in fish oil supplements, have anti-inflammatory properties and can support joint and heart health. If you don't consume fatty fish regularly, consider this supplement.

- Creatine: Creatine is one of the most researched and proven supplements for increasing muscle mass and strength. It enhances ATP production, which can lead to improved performance during high-intensity, short-duration activities like weightlifting.

- Caffeine: Caffeine can increase alertness and energy levels, potentially improving workout performance. However, its effects can vary from person to person, and excessive caffeine intake can lead to negative side effects.

It's crucial to approach supplements with caution. While they can provide benefits, they should never replace a balanced diet rich in whole foods. Supplements are meant to supplement your nutrition, not substitute it. Before adding any supplement to your regimen, consult with a healthcare professional to ensure it's safe and suitable for your specific needs and goals.

Potential Risks and Benefits

In the quest for bodybuilding glory, it's tempting to view supplements as shortcuts to success. However, it's essential to weigh the potential risks against the benefits, especially when it comes to the unregulated supplement industry.

Benefits:

Convenience: Supplements can be a convenient way to meet your nutritional needs, especially when you're on the go or need a quick protein fix post-workout.

Performance Enhancement: Some supplements, like creatine, caffeine, and BCAAs, may enhance performance and recovery, allowing you to push harder in the gym.

Micronutrient Insurance: Multivitamin supplements can provide a safety net to cover potential micronutrient gaps in your diet.

Risks:

Quality Control: The supplement industry is notorious for poor quality control and mislabeling. Not all supplements contain what they claim, and some may even be contaminated with harmful substances.

Dependency: Relying too heavily on supplements can lead to a dependency mindset, neglecting the importance of whole foods in your diet.

Side Effects: Some supplements can cause adverse side effects or interact with medications. It's crucial to research and consult a healthcare professional before adding them to your regimen.

Financial Cost: Quality supplements can be expensive, and the cost can add up quickly if you're not careful.

In the end, the decision to use supplements should be a calculated one, based on your individual needs, goals, and the potential benefits they offer. Remember that no supplement can replace the foundation of proper nutrition, consistency in training, and restorative sleep.

## Meal Planning and Timing

In the world of bodybuilding, where the pursuit of strength and aesthetics demands discipline and precision, the battle isn't just fought in the gym. It's waged on your plate, with every morsel of food, and every sip of liquid you consume. This chapter, "Meal Planning and Timing," is the blueprint for optimizing your nutrition strategy, ensuring that you fuel your body for peak performance and muscle growth without faltering in the face of dietary chaos.

The Importance of Meal Timing

In the battlefield of bodybuilding, timing is everything. It's not just about what you eat, but when you eat it. You wouldn't go to war without a strategy, and you shouldn't embark on your bodybuilding journey without a meal timing plan.

Pre-Workout Nutrition

Picture this: you're gearing up for a brutal training session, ready to unleash your inner beast on the weights. But there's an essential task at hand – fueling your body for the impending battle.

Pre-workout nutrition is your ticket to peak performance. It's about supplying your body with the right nutrients to ensure that you have the energy, focus, and strength needed to conquer your workout. The goal is simple: maximize your output in the gym, and you'll maximize your results.

Here's the breakdown:

Carbohydrates: Complex carbohydrates are your primary source of pre-workout fuel. They provide a steady release of energy to keep you going throughout your session. Think of them as the slow-burning fire that sustains your workout intensity.

Protein: While carbohydrates are the main event, protein plays a supporting role in pre-workout nutrition. It provides amino acids that help prevent muscle breakdown during your training session. It's like having body armor for your muscles.

Fats: Although fats aren't a primary focus of pre-workout nutrition, they can provide some sustained energy. However, keep fat intake moderate to avoid digestive discomfort during your workout.

Hydration: Hydration is non-negotiable. Dehydration can lead to decreased performance, fatigue, and even muscle cramps. Start your workout well-hydrated, and consider sipping on water or an electrolyte drink during your training.

The timing of your pre-workout meal or snack matters. You want to eat about 1 to 2 hours before hitting the gym, allowing your body to digest and absorb the nutrients effectively. If you're in a rush, a smaller snack 30 minutes before your workout can still provide a boost.

So, what does a pre-workout meal or snack look like in the real world?

Example Pre-Workout Meals:

- Grilled chicken breast with brown rice and steamed broccoli: A classic bodybuilder's choice, providing a balance of protein, complex carbs, and fiber for sustained energy.

- Greek yogurt with berries and a drizzle of honey: A quick and easy option rich in protein and carbohydrates.

- Oatmeal with sliced banana and a scoop of protein powder: A hearty meal with a blend of complex carbs and protein.

- Whole-grain toast with almond butter and a sprinkle of cinnamon: A simple yet effective choice that provides energy without being too heavy.

The key is to experiment and find what works best for you. Some people prefer a solid meal, while others opt for a light snack. Pay attention to how your body responds and adjust accordingly.

Intra-Workout Nutrition

During your intense training session, your muscles are working at full throttle, demanding fuel to sustain their performance. While you don't need a full-blown meal mid-workout, some strategic choices can keep your energy levels stable and support muscle recovery.

- Carbohydrate Sources: If your workout is exceptionally long or intense, consider sipping on a carbohydrate-based sports drink or consuming a carbohydrate gel to replenish glycogen stores and maintain energy levels.

- Amino Acids: Branched-Chain Amino Acids (BCAAs) or an essential amino acid supplement can help prevent muscle breakdown during extended workouts.

- Water: Stay hydrated throughout your workout. Dehydration can lead to decreased performance and muscle cramps.

- Intra-workout nutrition isn't always necessary for shorter training sessions, but it can be beneficial for marathon gym sessions or endurance training. Again, it's about customizing your strategy to match your specific needs.

- Post-Workout Nutrition: The Anabolic Window

You've just pushed your body to its limits, breaking down muscle fibers in the process. Now it's time for recovery, and post-workout nutrition is your secret weapon in the battle against muscle soreness and fatigue.

The post-workout period is often referred to as the "anabolic window." It's a window of opportunity when your muscles are primed for nutrient uptake, and the right choices can kick start the repair and growth process.

Here's what you need to know:

Protein: Post-workout, your muscles are hungry for protein. This is the time to provide them with the amino acids they need to rebuild and grow. Whey protein, due to its rapid digestion and absorption, is a popular choice, but other protein sources like lean meats, fish, eggs, or plant-based options work just as well.

Carbohydrates: Carbohydrates play a crucial role in post-workout nutrition as well. They replenish glycogen stores that were depleted during your workout and provide an insulin spike that can enhance protein uptake. Fast-digesting carbohydrates like white rice, potatoes, or simple sugars can be effective choices.

Hydration: Rehydrate with water or an electrolyte drink to replace fluids lost during your workout.

Timing: The post-workout meal or shake should be consumed ideally within 30 minutes to 2 hours after your workout. This timing can maximize the benefits of the anabolic window.

Example Post-Workout Meals:

- Grilled salmon with quinoa and steamed asparagus: A well-rounded meal providing protein, complex carbs, and essential nutrients.

- Protein shake with whey protein, a banana, and a tablespoon of honey: A quick and convenient option that hits the mark for protein and carbohydrates.

- Turkey sandwich on whole-grain bread with plenty of veggies: A balanced choice that combines protein, carbohydrates, and fiber.

- Vegan protein bowl with brown rice, tofu, and mixed vegetables: A plant-based option rich in protein and complex carbs.

Remember that your post-workout meal doesn't need to be overly complicated. The goal is to provide your body with the nutrients it needs for recovery and growth. Tailor your choices to your dietary preferences and sensitivities.

Meal Frequency: The 3-4 Hour Rule

In the world of bodybuilding, consistency is king. It's not just about what you eat but how often you eat. The 3-4 hour rule is a fundamental principle of meal frequency for bodybuilders. Here's how it works:

- Eat Every 3-4 Hours: You should aim to eat a meal or snack every 3-4 hours throughout the day. This consistent meal frequency helps maintain a steady supply of nutrients to support muscle growth and recovery.

- Prevents Muscle Breakdown: Eating regularly prevents your body from going into a catabolic state, where it breaks down muscle tissue for energy. By providing a constant stream of nutrients, you keep your muscles in an anabolic, or growth-promoting, state.

- Optimizes Nutrient Timing: The 3-4 hour rule aligns with the timing of your workouts. By having a meal or snack within a few hours of training, you ensure that your body has the necessary fuel to perform at its best during exercise. Post-workout, another meal or snack replenishes glycogen stores and provides the amino acids needed for muscle repair and growth.

- Balances Blood Sugar: Consistent meal frequency helps stabilize blood sugar levels. Sharp spikes and crashes in blood sugar can lead to cravings, mood swings, and energy slumps. By eating every 3-4 hours, you maintain steady energy levels and reduce the risk of overindulging in unhealthy snacks.

- Supports Metabolism: Regular meals and snacks keep your metabolism revved up. Your body burns calories while digesting and processing food, and frequent eating helps maintain this calorie-burning process throughout the day.

- Prevents Overeating: When you allow too much time between meals, you're more likely to become ravenous and overeat during your next meal. By eating every 3-4 hours, you can better control portion sizes and make healthier food choices.

- Promotes Hydration: Meal frequency also encourages regular hydration. Many bodybuilders forget that water intake is as crucial as food. By eating frequently, you're reminded to stay hydrated, supporting digestion and overall health.

- Creates Routine and Structure: Consistency in meal frequency creates a structured daily routine. This structure can help you plan your workouts, meals, and other activities, making it easier to stay on track with your bodybuilding goals.

- Now, while the 3-4 hour rule is a solid guideline, it's essential to adapt it to your individual needs and schedule. Some people may thrive with more frequent meals, while others may find three main meals and a couple of snacks to be sufficient. The key is to listen to your body and ensure you're meeting your daily calorie and nutrient requirements.

- Incorporate lean proteins, complex carbohydrates, and healthy fats into your meals and snacks to support muscle growth, energy, and overall health. Remember that portion control is vital, even when eating frequently, to avoid excessive calorie intake.

- Consistency is the cornerstone of success in bodybuilding. Whether you're in the bulking or cutting phase, adhering to a regular meal frequency is a non-negotiable part of your nutrition strategy. Embrace the 3-4 hour rule as a fundamental principle in your bodybuilding journey, and watch how it contributes to your progress, one meal at a time.

# Nutritional Strategies for Bulking and Cutting

The chapter at hand, "Nutritional Strategies for Bulking and Cutting," is the unwavering blueprint for sculpting your physique, whether you're adding mass or chiseling it to perfection. It's not about following the latest fad or blindly cramming calories; it's about calculated and ruthless nutrition tactics that will propel you towards your bodybuilding goals.

The Bulking Phase: Building the Foundation of Power

Bulking isn't about mindlessly gorging on everything in sight. It's a calculated and strategic approach to building muscle and strength. In this phase, you're in a caloric surplus, consuming more calories than your body burns. The goal is to provide your muscles with an abundance of nutrients to fuel growth, repair, and recovery.

- Caloric Surplus: To bulk effectively, you need a surplus of calories. But don't take it as a license to eat everything in sight. The surplus should be controlled, ensuring that the additional calories go towards muscle growth, not fat storage.

- Macronutrient Ratios: While your macros (protein, carbohydrates, and fats) will largely remain the same, you may adjust the ratios slightly. Protein remains crucial for muscle repair, while carbohydrates provide the energy needed to fuel those intense workouts. Healthy fats should be a part of your diet, but their role is supportive, not primary.

- Protein: Aim to maintain a protein intake of around 1.2 to 2.2 grams per kilogram of body weight. Protein is your muscle's best friend, ensuring you recover and grow optimally during the bulking phase.

- Carbohydrates: Carbs should make up a significant portion of your diet, providing energy for your workouts and aiding in muscle recovery. Complex carbohydrates are your allies, delivering sustained energy without the sugar crashes.

- Fats: Healthy fats are essential for overall health, including hormone production, but keep them in moderation. They're supplementary, helping you meet your caloric needs.

- Meal Timing: The 3-4 hour meal frequency rule still applies. Consistent nutrient intake keeps your body in an anabolic state, conducive to muscle growth.

Examples of Bulking Meals:

- Grilled chicken breast with quinoa, roasted sweet potatoes, and a side of steamed broccoli: A balanced meal providing protein, complex carbs, and fiber.

- Whole-grain pasta with lean ground beef and a tomato-based sauce: A hearty meal rich in protein and complex carbs.

- Protein shake with whey protein, oats, banana, and almond butter: A nutrient-dense option for an additional calorie boost.

The Cutting Phase: Chiseling Your Masterpiece

Once you've built the foundation of muscle mass during the bulking phase, it's time to reveal the masterpiece beneath. The cutting phase is all about shedding body fat while preserving your hard-earned muscle. It's a meticulous dance between calorie restriction and macronutrient optimization.

Caloric Deficit: Cutting involves consuming fewer calories than your body burns, creating a caloric deficit.

However, it's crucial to strike a balance – too much of a deficit can lead to muscle loss.

Protein: Your protein intake remains high during cutting to preserve muscle mass. Aim for the same protein range as in the bulking phase.

Carbohydrates: Carbs should still be a part of your diet but may be adjusted downward. Focus on complex carbs to keep you feeling full and energized.

Fats: Healthy fats remain in your diet, as they support overall health and hormone balance. They can also aid in satiety during calorie restriction.

Meal Timing: The 3-4 hour rule continues to be your guide during the cutting phase. Consistency in meal frequency is vital to maintain muscle and curb cravings.

Examples of Cutting Meals:

- Grilled salmon with a side of quinoa and steamed asparagus: A lean protein source combined with complex carbs and fiber for satiety.

- Salad with grilled chicken, mixed greens, and a vinaigrette dressing: A low-calorie, high-protein meal that keeps you feeling full.

- Stir-fried tofu with broccoli and brown rice: A plant-based option rich in protein and complex carbs.

Cardio and Training: Cardio can be a valuable tool during the cutting phase to enhance calorie burning. High-intensity interval training (HIIT) is particularly effective for fat loss. However, don't overdo it, as excessive cardio can lead to muscle loss.

Supplements: During cutting, supplements like BCAAs and whey protein can help preserve muscle and manage cravings. Remember, though, supplements are a complement to your diet, not a replacement.

Hydration: Staying hydrated is crucial during cutting, as thirst can sometimes be mistaken for hunger. Drink plenty of water throughout the day.

Tracking Progress: Keep a close eye on your progress during the cutting phase. Regular assessments of body composition, such as body fat percentage and muscle mass, can help you fine-tune your approach.

Cheat Meals: While discipline is essential, occasional cheat meals can be a mental relief and help prevent binging. Keep them controlled and don't let them derail your progress.

Cycling: Some bodybuilders employ calorie cycling during the cutting phase, alternating between higher and lower-calorie days. This approach can help prevent metabolic adaptation and maintain muscle.

Refeeding: Periodic refeeding days, where you temporarily increase your calorie intake, can help reset hormone levels and alleviate some of the metabolic slowdown associated with prolonged calorie restriction.

The key to success in the cutting phase is discipline and consistency. It's not an easy journey, and it demands mental fortitude, but the results are worth the sacrifice. Cutting is about revealing the masterpiece you've sculpted during bulking, and the sharper your tools, the more impeccable your creation will be.

# Specialized Diets for Bodybuilders

Nutrition is the unsung hero that separates the champions from the rest. This chapter, "Specialized Diets for Bodybuilders," isn't about quick fixes or trendy diets; it's about ruthless and calculated approaches to nutrition that can take your physique to the next level. If you're ready to push your limits and sculpt your body into a work of art, read on.

Ketogenic Diet: Carving out the Fat

The ketogenic diet, often dubbed "keto," has gained notoriety for its remarkable ability to shed body fat like a hot knife through butter. This high-fat, low-carb diet is a weapon of choice for bodybuilders looking to get leaner while preserving muscle mass.

In a ketogenic diet:

- Carbohydrates are severely restricted: Typically, carbs make up only about 5-10% of total daily calories. This restriction forces your body to rely on fat for fuel instead of glucose from carbs.

- Fats take the spotlight: Approximately 70-80% of your daily calories come from healthy fats like avocados, nuts, seeds, and oils. These fats become the primary energy source.

- Protein remains moderate: Protein intake hovers around 15-20% of daily calories. It's sufficient to support muscle maintenance and growth.

The ketogenic diet induces a state called ketosis, where your body starts producing ketones from fat breakdown. Ketones serve as an alternative fuel source for your muscles and brain. During this process, your body becomes incredibly efficient at burning stored fat for energy, making it an excellent choice for cutting phases.

However, the keto diet isn't a walk in the park. It demands strict adherence, and the initial transition can be mentally and physically challenging as your body adapts to the absence of carbs. It's not a long-term solution, but when used strategically during cutting phases, it can yield remarkable results in shedding body fat while preserving muscle.

Cyclical Ketogenic Diet: The Best of Both Worlds

For those who crave carbohydrates, the cyclical ketogenic diet (CKD) offers a compromise. CKD involves cycling between periods of strict keto and short "carb-loading" phases.

Here's how it works:

- Keto Phase: During this phase, which can last anywhere from 5 to 6 days, you follow a strict ketogenic diet, similar to what was described earlier. Your carb intake is minimal.

- Carb-Loading Phase: This is the break you've been waiting for. On this day (or sometimes two days), you load up on carbs, sometimes exceeding your daily calorie needs. This carb influx refills muscle glycogen stores and provides a mental and physical boost.

CKD offers the metabolic benefits of ketosis while providing periodic relief from carb restriction. It's a strategy favored by some bodybuilders to enjoy the best of both worlds – the fat-shredding power of keto and the muscle-sparing properties of carb refeeds.

Intermittent Fasting: Fasting for Gains

Intermittent fasting (IF) is a nutritional strategy that's gained popularity in recent years, thanks to its simplicity and potential health benefits. For bodybuilders, it can be a valuable tool for managing calorie intake, improving insulin sensitivity, and supporting fat loss.

IF involves cycling between periods of fasting and eating. Here are some common IF approaches:

- 16/8 Method: This method involves fasting for 16 hours each day and limiting your eating window to 8 hours. Most people achieve this by skipping breakfast and eating their first meal around noon.

- 5:2 Method: In this approach, you eat normally for five days of the week and limit calorie intake to around 500-600 calories on the remaining two days.

- Eat-Stop-Eat: With this method, you fast for a full 24 hours once or twice a week. For example, you might eat dinner at 7 pm one day and not eat again until 7 pm the following day.

- Alternate-Day Fasting: This approach involves alternating between days of regular eating and days of fasting or consuming very few calories.

Intermittent fasting isn't about restricting specific food groups or macronutrients; it's about controlling when you eat. During the fasting period, your body taps into stored fat for energy, potentially aiding in fat loss. It can also improve insulin sensitivity, which is beneficial for overall health and muscle growth.

However, IF may not be suitable for everyone, especially those with specific dietary requirements or training schedules. It's essential to tailor the fasting approach to your individual needs and goals.

Vegetarian and Vegan Diets: Plant-Powered Gains

Contrary to the misconception that bodybuilding relies solely on animal protein, vegetarian and vegan diets can also be powerful tools for muscle growth and strength. With careful planning and strategic food choices, plant-powered bodybuilders can achieve remarkable results.

Here's how it's done:

- Protein Sources: Plant-based protein sources become the cornerstone of your diet. These include tofu, tempeh, seitan, legumes (such as lentils, chickpeas, and black beans), and plant-based protein powders. Nuts and seeds are also excellent protein sources.

- Amino Acid Balance: To ensure you're getting all the essential amino acids, it's crucial to diversify your protein sources. Combining different plant proteins, like beans and rice, can help achieve a balanced amino acid profile.

- Iron-Rich Foods: Plant-based diets can provide plenty of iron through foods like dark leafy greens, fortified cereals, and legumes. Iron is essential for oxygen transport, which is crucial during workouts.

- B12 Supplementation: Vitamin B12 is primarily found in animal products, so many vegetarians and vegans need to supplement or consume B12-fortified foods to avoid deficiencies.

- Caloric Surplus: To build muscle, you'll still need a caloric surplus, just like any other bodybuilder. This means consuming more calories than you burn to support muscle growth.

Vegetarian and vegan bodybuilders can enjoy the same benefits as their omnivorous counterparts – increased muscle mass, strength, and improved overall health. With proper planning and a keen eye on nutrient intake, plant-powered bodybuilders can thrive in the gym and on the stage.

Carb Cycling: Timing Your Carbs for Gains

Carb cycling is a strategic approach to nutrition that involves alternating between high-carb and low-carb days. It's a favorite among bodybuilders for optimizing energy levels, supporting muscle growth, and managing body fat.

The premise of carb cycling is straightforward:

- **High-Carb Days:** On these days, you increase your carbohydrate intake to support intense workouts and refuel muscle glycogen stores. High-carb days are often aligned with your most grueling

# Staying Hydrated

In bodybuilding, two crucial elements often take a back seat: hydration and progress monitoring. Neglecting these can be the Achilles' heel that undermines your journey to sculpting the ultimate physique. In this chapter, we'll delve into the unsung heroes of bodybuilding – staying hydrated and monitoring progress. No fluff, no frills, just raw knowledge to elevate your game.

Hydration: The Overlooked Game Changer

Water is the unsung hero of your bodybuilding arsenal. While you're busy counting reps and tracking macros, hydration often slips through the cracks. Yet, it's one of the most critical components of your success. Without proper hydration, your body can't perform at its peak, and your gains will suffer.

The Importance of Hydration

Picture this: you're in the midst of an intense workout, beads of sweat pouring down your face, and your muscles pushing to their limit. Every movement is a testament to your dedication. But there's an often-underestimated factor at play – your hydration status.

Hydration is not just about quenching your thirst; it's about ensuring that your body functions optimally. Here's why it matters:

- Muscle Function: Dehydration can lead to muscle cramps and decreased muscle contractions, hampering your performance.

- Temperature Regulation: Sweating is your body's cooling mechanism. Without sufficient water, you risk overheating, which can be dangerous during intense workouts.

- Energy Levels: Even mild dehydration can lead to fatigue and reduced energy levels, making it harder to push through your training sessions.

- Recovery: Proper hydration is essential for post-workout recovery. It helps transport nutrients to your muscles, aiding in repair and growth.

- Cognitive Function: Dehydration can impair focus and cognitive function, affecting your workout intensity and form.

How Much Water Do You Need?

The age-old advice of drinking eight 8-ounce glasses of water a day is a good starting point for the average person. However, bodybuilders often have greater hydration needs due to their intense training regimens and increased sweat rates.

A more personalized approach is to calculate your water needs based on your body weight. As a general guideline, aim for about 30-35 milliliters of water per kilogram of body weight per day. For example, if you weigh 70 kilograms (154 pounds), you'd need approximately 2,100 to 2,450 milliliters of water daily.

Keep in mind that individual factors like climate, activity level, and sweat rate can affect your hydration requirements. On intense workout days, you may need to drink even more to compensate for fluid loss.

Signs of Dehydration

Detecting dehydration early is crucial to prevent its detrimental effects. Here are some common signs to watch out for:

- Thirst: The most apparent signal that your body needs water.

- Dark Urine: Dark yellow or amber-colored urine is a sign of dehydration. Your urine should be pale yellow.

- Dry Mouth and Skin: Dry or sticky feeling in your mouth and skin can indicate dehydration.

- Fatigue: If you feel unusually tired during your workout or throughout the day, it could be due to dehydration.

- Headache: Dehydration can trigger headaches and migraines.

- Muscle Cramps: Frequent muscle cramps, especially during exercise, may be a sign of inadequate hydration.

Strategies for Staying Hydrated

Now that you understand the importance of hydration let's dive into some strategies to ensure you stay adequately hydrated:

- Drink Throughout the Day: Don't wait until you're thirsty to start drinking. Sip water consistently throughout the day.

- Pre-Workout Hydration: Drink a glass of water about 2 hours before your workout to ensure you start your training session well-hydrated.

- During Workout: Sip on water or an electrolyte drink during your workout, especially if it's intense or lengthy. Electrolyte drinks can help replace lost minerals through sweat.

- Post-Workout Rehydration: After your workout, rehydrate with water or a recovery drink to replace fluid losses.

- Monitor Urine Color: Keep an eye on the color of your urine. If it's pale yellow, you're likely well-hydrated. Dark yellow or amber urine is a sign to drink more water.

- Consider Your Environment: Hot and humid conditions can increase sweat rates, so you'll need to drink more to compensate.

- Electrolytes: If you're sweating excessively, especially in a hot climate, consider incorporating electrolyte drinks or foods high in electrolytes, like bananas or coconut water, into your regimen.

Hydration is the foundation of your bodybuilding journey. It's not an option; it's a necessity. Neglecting it can undermine your hard work and dedication in the gym. So, remember to drink up, even when the iron is calling your name.

## Monitoring Progress: Your North Star

Progress isn't just a goal; it's the guiding light that keeps you on track. Yet, many aspiring bodybuilders stumble in the dark, not knowing how to navigate their journey.

That's where progress monitoring comes in – your North Star in the constellation of gains.

Why Monitor Progress

Imagine setting sail on a treacherous sea without a compass or map. You'd be lost in the vastness, drifting aimlessly. The same holds for bodybuilding. Monitoring your progress is your compass, guiding you through the turbulent waters of training and nutrition.

Here's why it matters:

- Motivation: Tracking your progress can be incredibly motivating. It allows you to see the fruits of your labor and provides a sense of achievement.

- Adjustments: Without monitoring, you're flying blind. Progress tracking helps you identify what's working and what isn't, allowing you to make necessary adjustments to your training and nutrition.

- Plateau Prevention: It's not uncommon to hit plateaus in your bodybuilding journey. Progress monitoring helps you recognize when progress stalls so you can pivot and keep moving forward.

- Accountability: When you're tracking your progress, you're less likely to skip workouts or deviate from your nutrition plan. It creates a sense of accountability to your goals.

What to Monitor

Progress monitoring goes beyond simply stepping on a scale. While body weight is one factor, it's far from the only one. Here's what you should be tracking:

- Body Weight: Your weight can provide insights into changes in muscle mass and body fat. However, it's not the sole indicator of progress, as fluctuations can occur due to various factors.

- Body Measurements: Tracking measurements of key areas like chest, waist, hips, arms, and legs can give you a more comprehensive view of your body's transformation. These measurements can help you identify changes in specific muscle groups and areas where you might be losing fat.

- Body Fat Percentage: Measuring your body fat percentage is crucial for understanding how your body composition is evolving. It's a more accurate reflection of progress than body weight alone, as it accounts for changes in muscle and fat.

- Strength and Performance: Keep a close eye on your strength and performance in the gym. Are you lifting heavier weights, completing more reps, or improving your workout intensity?

These improvements signal muscle growth and increased fitness levels.

- Energy Levels: Your energy levels are a valuable indicator of your overall health. As your nutrition and training plan progress, you should experience increased energy and endurance during workouts and throughout the day.

- Recovery and Soreness: Pay attention to how quickly you recover from workouts and the level of soreness you experience. Improved recovery and reduced soreness can indicate that your nutrition plan is supporting muscle repair and growth.

- Mood and Mental Clarity: Nutrition doesn't just affect your body; it has a significant impact on your mind. Monitor changes in mood, mental clarity, and focus. A well-balanced diet can enhance your cognitive function and overall well-being.

- Sleep Quality: Adequate sleep is essential for recovery and muscle growth. Track your sleep quality and duration. Improved sleep patterns are a positive sign that your nutrition and training are on the right track.

- Skin Health: The condition of your skin can also reflect your nutritional status. Healthy, clear skin can be a sign of a well-balanced diet with adequate hydration.

- Hunger and Appetite: Pay attention to your hunger and appetite cues. A well-structured nutrition plan should help regulate your appetite and reduce cravings for unhealthy foods.

- Digestive Health: Digestive issues can hinder nutrient absorption. Monitor your digestive health and make adjustments to your diet if you experience discomfort, bloating, or irregularity.

- While these indicators are essential for tracking progress, remember that changes won't happen overnight. Patience and consistency are your allies on this journey. Use these markers to make informed adjustments to your nutrition plan and training regimen as you work toward your bodybuilding goals. The path to mastery is marked by these small steps and incremental improvements, and every bit of progress is a step closer to the body you're sculpting.

## Common Mistakes and Pitfalls

In the relentless pursuit of the perfect physique, where sweat and iron are your constant companions, there's little room for error. Yet, even the most dedicated bodybuilders can stumble and fall prey to common mistakes and pitfalls along the way. In this chapter, we'll expose these pitfalls, not to dwell on them, but to arm you with the knowledge to sidestep these traps and keep forging ahead.

Neglecting Proper Warm-Ups and Cool-Downs

Picture this: you walk into the gym, fueled with determination, ready to conquer the weights. You head straight to the squat rack, load up the bar, and dive into your working sets. Sounds familiar? It's a common scenario, but it's also a recipe for disaster.

The Mistake: Neglecting proper warm-ups and cool-downs.

Why It's a Pitfall: Failing to warm up adequately can increase the risk of injuries and reduce your performance during your workout. Conversely, skipping a cool-down can lead to delayed onset muscle soreness (DOMS) and hinder recovery.

The Solution: Prioritize your warm-up and cool-down routines. Start with 5-10 minutes of light aerobic activity to increase blood flow to your muscles. Follow it with dynamic stretching or mobility exercises to prepare your body for the workout ahead. After your workout, dedicate another 5-10 minutes to static stretching and foam rolling to aid recovery.

Overtraining and Under-Recovery

In the pursuit of gains, more is not always better. Many bodybuilders fall victim to the belief that relentless training and minimal rest will accelerate progress. However, this approach can lead to a vicious cycle of overtraining and under-recovery.

The Mistake: Overtraining and neglecting the importance of recovery.

Why It's a Pitfall: Overtraining can lead to fatigue, decreased performance, increased risk of injuries, and even hormonal imbalances. It hampers your body's ability to repair and grow muscle.

The Solution: Prioritize rest and recovery as much as your training sessions. Ensure you're getting adequate sleep, as it's during slumber that your body performs its most significant recovery and repair work. Implement planned deload weeks in your training program to allow your body to recuperate fully. Listen to your body; if you're feeling excessively fatigued or experiencing chronic soreness, it's a sign to ease up and prioritize recovery.

Ignoring Proper Form

In the world of bodybuilding, lifting heavy is a badge of honor. However, this pursuit of weightlifting supremacy can often come at the expense of proper form and technique.

The Mistake: Ignoring proper form and prioritizing lifting heavier weights.

Why It's a Pitfall: Neglecting form can lead to injuries and limit muscle activation. It shifts the focus from targeted muscle groups to secondary muscles, reducing the effectiveness of your exercises.

The Solution: Prioritize proper form above all else. Focus on controlled, full-range-of-motion repetitions. Reduce the weight if needed to maintain good form. If you're unsure about your technique, seek guidance from a qualified trainer or use mirrors to visually assess your form during exercises.

Neglecting Nutrient Timing

Nutrition is the lifeblood of bodybuilding, and timing plays a crucial role in optimizing your results. Yet, many bodybuilders overlook the significance of nutrient timing, missing out on the full potential of their nutrition strategy.

The Mistake: Neglecting nutrient timing, such as pre-workout and post-workout nutrition.

Why It's a Pitfall: Timing your nutrients strategically can enhance workout performance, muscle recovery, and growth. Neglecting this aspect can leave gains on the table.

The Solution: Prioritize pre-workout and post-workout nutrition. Consume a balanced meal or snack 1-2 hours before your workout, focusing on a combination of carbohydrates and protein. After your workout, have a post-workout meal or shake within 30 minutes to 2 hours, emphasizing protein and fast-digesting carbohydrates to kickstart recovery.

Excessive Supplementation

The supplement industry is a billion-dollar business, and it's easy to fall into the trap of believing that a cabinet full of pills and powders will be the key to your success.

The Mistake: Relying too heavily on supplements.

Why It's a Pitfall: Supplements are meant to complement your diet, not replace it. Depending on supplements can lead to nutrient imbalances and financial strain.

The Solution: Prioritize whole foods as the foundation of your nutrition. Supplements should be used strategically to fill gaps in your diet, not as a primary source of nutrients. Focus on essentials like protein powder, creatine, and branched-chain amino acids (BCAAs), but don't neglect a well-balanced diet.

Inconsistent Tracking

In the world of bodybuilding, consistency is king. Whether it's tracking your workouts, nutrition, or progress, inconsistency can lead to stagnation.

The Mistake: Inconsistent tracking of workouts, nutrition, and progress.

Why It's a Pitfall: Inconsistency makes it challenging to identify what's working and what isn't. It hinders your ability to make informed adjustments to your training and nutrition plan.

The Solution: Prioritize consistency in tracking. Keep a detailed workout journal, recording exercises, sets, reps, and weights. Track your daily nutrition intake, including macros and calories. Take regular progress photos and measurements to monitor changes in your physique. This data will be invaluable in fine-tuning your approach and ensuring steady progress.

Neglecting Mobility and Flexibility

In the quest for muscle and strength, flexibility and mobility are often disregarded. However, these aspects are crucial for injury prevention and optimal performance.

The Mistake: Neglecting mobility and flexibility training.

Why It's a Pitfall: Poor mobility and flexibility can lead to imbalances, reduced range of motion, and an increased risk of injuries. It can also hinder your ability to perform exercises with proper form.

The Solution: Prioritize mobility and flexibility exercises in your routine. Include dynamic stretches and mobility drills in your warm-up to prepare your muscles and joints for exercise. Dedicate time to static stretching and foam rolling in your cool-down to enhance flexibility and aid recovery.

Progress isn't always a linear path. You'll encounter setbacks, challenges, and moments of self-doubt. However, by learning from the common mistakes and pitfalls that many bodybuilders face, you can navigate your journey with greater confidence and success. Remember, it's not about avoiding these pitfalls entirely; it's about recognizing them, learning from them, and using them as stepping stones toward your ultimate goal: mastery of your body and your craft.

## Example Meal Plans

In this chapter, we won't delve into the intricacies of theory or dabble in the hypothetical; we'll cut through the noise and lay bare the practicality of nutrition mastery with concrete example meal plans. No frills, no fluff, just the battle-tested fuel that will propel you closer to your bodybuilding goals.

Meal Plan 1: Fuel for Bulking

Bulking isn't an invitation for reckless eating; it's a calculated assault on muscle growth. Here's a meal plan that provides the sustenance needed to add mass without sacrificing quality.

Meal 1: Breakfast

- Scrambled Eggs: 3 large eggs cooked in olive oil for healthy fats and protein.

- Whole-Grain Toast: 2 slices for complex carbs and fiber.

- Spinach and Tomato: A side of veggies for vitamins and minerals.

Meal 2: Mid-Morning Snack

- Greek Yogurt: 1 cup for protein and probiotics.

- Mixed Berries: A handful for antioxidants and flavor.

Meal 3: Lunch

- Grilled Chicken Breast: 6 ounces for lean protein.

- Quinoa: 1 cup for complex carbs and fiber.

- Steamed Broccoli: A side of greens for nutrients.

Meal 4: Pre-Workout

- Protein Shake: 1 scoop of whey protein for fast-digesting amino acids.

- Banana: A quick source of energy.

Meal 5: Post-Workout

- Salmon: 6 ounces for protein and healthy fats.

- Brown Rice: 1 cup for sustained energy.

- Asparagus: A side of greens for vitamins and fiber.

Meal 6: Dinner

- Lean Beef Steak: 6 ounces for protein and iron.

- Sweet Potatoes: 1 cup for complex carbs and beta-carotene.

- Mixed Vegetables: A side of colorful veggies for vitamins.

Meal 7: Evening Snack

- Cottage Cheese: 1 cup for casein protein (slow-digesting).

- Almonds: A small handful for healthy fats.

Meal Plan 2: Precision for Cutting

Cutting is about sculpting your masterpiece by shedding excess body fat while preserving muscle. This meal plan provides the precision needed to reveal the chiseled physique beneath.

Meal 1: Breakfast

- Oatmeal: 1 cup for complex carbs and fiber.

- Egg Whites: 4 egg whites for protein.

- Spinach: A handful for added nutrients.

Meal 2: Mid-Morning Snack

- Protein Shake: 1 scoop of whey protein.

- Almonds: A small handful for healthy fats.

Meal 3: Lunch

- Grilled Turkey Breast: 6 ounces for lean protein.

- Quinoa Salad: 1 cup for complex carbs and fiber.

- Mixed Greens: A generous portion for vitamins.

Meal 4: Pre-Workout

- Greek Yogurt: 1 cup for protein.

- Berries: A handful for antioxidants.

Meal 5: Post-Workout

- Chicken Breast: 6 ounces for lean protein.

- Brown Rice: 1 cup for complex carbs.

- Broccoli: A side of greens for vitamins and fiber.

Meal 6: Dinner

- Salmon: 6 ounces for protein and healthy fats.

- Asparagus: A side of greens for nutrients.

- Quinoa: 1/2 cup for additional carbs.

Meal 7: Evening Snack

- Cottage Cheese: 1 cup for casein protein.

- Walnuts: A small handful for healthy fats.

Meal Plan 3: Vegetarian Power

Contrary to the misconception that bodybuilding relies solely on animal protein, a vegetarian meal plan can provide the power needed for muscle growth and strength.

Meal 1: Breakfast

- Scrambled Tofu: Tofu cooked with veggies for protein and nutrients.

- Whole-Grain Toast: 2 slices for complex carbs.

- Spinach and Tomato: A side of greens for vitamins.

Meal 2: Mid-Morning Snack

- Greek Yogurt: 1 cup for protein.

- Mixed Berries: A handful for antioxidants.

Meal 3: Lunch

- Tempeh Stir-Fry: Tempeh with mixed vegetables for protein and fiber.

- Brown Rice: 1 cup for complex carbs.

Meal 4: Pre-Workout

- Protein Shake: 1 scoop of plant-based protein.

- Banana: A quick source of energy.

Meal 5: Post-Workout

- Chickpea Salad: Chickpeas with veggies for protein and fiber.

- Quinoa: 1/2 cup for additional carbs.

Meal 6: Dinner

- Lentil Curry: Lentils cooked with spices and served with brown rice for protein and complex carbs.

- Mixed Vegetables: A side of greens for vitamins.

Meal 7: Evening Snack

- Cottage Cheese: 1 cup for casein protein.

- Almonds: A small handful for healthy fats.

These meal plans are not set in stone but serve as templates to demonstrate the practicality of a balanced nutrition strategy. The key to success is consistency and adaptability. Tailor your meals to your preferences and dietary requirements while adhering to your macro and calorie targets. Remember, nutrition mastery is about the relentless pursuit of your bodybuilding goals, one meal at a time.

# Emerging Trends And Technologies

Emerging trends and technologies in variable resistance training are shaping the future of fitness, offering innovative approaches and enhanced efficiency in workouts. One of the significant trends is the increasing use of smart technology in training equipment. Smart resistance machines and equipment are being developed, which can automatically adjust resistance based on the user's performance, strength level, and even biometric feedback. These smart machines use algorithms to determine the optimal resistance for each exercise phase, ensuring maximum efficiency and safety.

Another trend is the integration of virtual and augmented reality in training programs. These technologies offer immersive experiences that can make workouts more engaging and interactive. For instance, virtual reality setups can simulate various training environments, providing real-time feedback and adjustments in resistance based on the user's performance. This approach not only enhances the training experience but also aids in maintaining correct form and technique.

Wearable technology is also playing a significant role in variable resistance training. Wearables like smartwatches and fitness trackers are increasingly being used to monitor performance, track progress, and even control resistance levels on compatible training equipment. These devices can provide immediate feedback on training intensity, muscle engagement, and overall workout effectiveness, allowing for more personalized and adaptive training programs.

The use of artificial intelligence (AI) in creating personalized training routines is gaining popularity. AI algorithms can analyze an individual's training data and provide recommendations for workout adjustments, including changes in variable resistance levels to optimize training outcomes. This personalization can lead to more effective workouts tailored to the user's specific fitness goals and needs.

Additionally, there is a growing emphasis on incorporating variable resistance training in rehabilitation and physiotherapy. Advanced equipment that can precisely control resistance levels is being used to aid in recovery from injuries and improve mobility. This equipment can adjust the resistance to match the patient's rehabilitation stage, providing a gradual and controlled strengthening pathway.

Finally, the development of more portable and affordable variable resistance equipment is making this type of training more accessible. Portable resistance bands with adjustable tension, compact spring-loaded equipment, and lightweight hydraulic devices are becoming popular among home users and those who prefer to train outside traditional gym settings.

## Conclusion

The concept of Variable Resistance Training (VRT) marks a significant departure from traditional weight training methods. In contrast to the constant load offered by traditional weights, VRT introduces a dynamic element to resistance. This means that the level of resistance changes throughout the exercise movement. Traditional weight training, with its constant resistance, has been the standard for strength and fitness for many years. It offers a straightforward approach where the load does not change during the exercise, thus providing a consistent challenge to the muscles throughout the movement.

However, this constancy can also be a limitation, as it might not align with the natural strength curve of muscles, which varies at different points in their range of motion. VRT addresses this by varying the resistance, thereby matching the body's natural strength fluctuations. This variation can lead to more effective muscle activation, as it challenges muscles more significantly at their strongest points while reducing the risk of injury by easing the load at weaker points.

Furthermore, VRT can help overcome the plateaus commonly experienced in traditional weight training, as the muscles are continually challenged by the changing resistance. This innovative approach to strength training offers a potentially more efficient and safer way to exercise, making it a compelling alternative to traditional methods.